WHO**STOLE**MY**BODY**

The Right Way to **Lose Weight**

WHO**STOLE**MY**BODY**

The Right Way to Lose Weight

MICHAEL ROMIG

Niche Pressworks

Who Stole My Body?

978-1-946533-81-4 (paperback)

978-1-946533-75-3 (ebook)

This book is not intended for the treatment or prevention of disease, nor is it a replacement for seeking medical treatment or professional fitness advice. Do not start any nutrition or physical activity program without first consulting your physician. The use of this program is at the sole risk of the reader. The author is neither responsible nor liable for any harm or injury resulting from the use of this program.

For permission to reprint portions of this content or bulk purchases, contact PG FIT, LLC at 832-303-7004.

Published by Niche Pressworks; http://NichePressworks.com

Dedication

I would like to dedicate this book to all of our clients at PG FIT, and to all of the clients that I have had the opportunity to work with over the years. If it weren't for you, then I would have never become the fitness professional I am today. You have taught me so many valuable life lessons and have helped me to learn, grow, and fall in love with the fitness industry. There is truly no greater calling than to be a personal trainer and to serve others.

Acknowledgements

I would first and foremost like to thank my wife, Katie, my son, Ben, and my family. To Katie and Ben, thank you for allowing me to pursue my passion for helping other people and for always being there. Thank you, Mom and Dad, for being such wonderful parents. I hope that I can set as good of an example for Ben as you have for me. To Tammie, Arianna, and Skyla, I'm always there if you need me. To Travis, Ashley, and Amelia, I hope to visit with you again really soon. To Trevor, I am always thinking about you and wishing you the best. To Clinton, we will have to go to an Astros game soon. I would also like to thank my in-laws. Diane, I always appreciate our deep conversations. Jim and Gloria, we are thinking about you and wishing you good health. To Arlene, Lillian, and Will, we are always here if you need anything. Without all of your love and support, this book would have never been possible. We have had our fair share of trials and tribulations over the last few years, but we have always persevered through them and will continue to do so.

I would also like to thank Casey, for being in the trenches with me every day. Thank you for your dedication and commitment to helping our clients accomplish their health and fitness goals. The best part of what we do is the people we get to work with. You truly inspire me to be the best person I possibly can be and to have a servant-like attitude.

Lastly, I would also like to thank all of the many personal trainers and coaches that I have worked with and mentored over the years. I have learned so much from you, but the most important lesson I have learned is that together, we can truly make a difference in our communities.

Contents

Foreword

I remember the moment I met Michael Romig. It was years ago, and I was speaking at an event. One of my friends said, "You have to meet this guy. His name is Michael, and he's a health and fitness expert." When I went over to meet him, he was welcoming and had such a cool vibe about him. Michael is super fit and strong, but what impressed me most about him was his heart and love for people.

As we talked throughout the day, Michael shared his vision for PG Fit and the difference he wanted to make in the world. He was focused on helping people truly understand their body and live their highest quality of life.

I often think about that day and how the vision Michael shared is now a reality. What's so exciting is that you're about to transform your health and fitness with his program.

We live in a world that is full of false health and fitness hype, and it's difficult to know what's authentic. And this is why I'm so excited for you. Michael's program is going to take you on an adventure that will empower you to own your fitness and food so that you can permanently achieve your goals.

What impresses me most about his program is how realistic it is. I'm a dad, husband, and entrepreneur. I live a busy life, and I assume you do too. Michael is also a dad, husband, and of course, health and fitness expert. He lives what he teaches and has spent the last twenty years perfecting his program with his thousands of clients to ensure YOU will win every step of the way.

Michael's techniques and strategies will apply to your everyday life and not only strengthen your body to the core, but also help your family. As I've traveled the world, the lessons I've learned from Michael's program have made an enormous difference by helping me build strength while maintaining high energy levels and feeling great.

As you start your amazing journey with Michael, I suggest you remember three things …

First, have fun! Michael's program is all about making health and fitness a way of life, and the best way to accomplish that is by having fun with his cutting-edge strategies.

Second, live his program with a friend. You'll get three times better results by taking on each day with a buddy. Friends help each other have fun, share new ideas, and provide necessary support during the tough days.

Third, be a part of Michael's PG Fit community. Once you're having fun and you have a buddy, it's time to expand your horizon and connect with thousands of other people experiencing the same health and fitness transformation you are. These connections and the support they provide create a foundation and ensure you will WIN forever with your health.

Okay, enough from me! It's time for you to start your next health and fitness chapter and begin your incredible journey with Michael.

Michael will lead you through each step of the process, building maximum momentum within each page. And as a huge fan and member of the PG Fit community, I can't wait to see your transformation and hear the power of your story. The community is cheering you on like the Champion you are!

Massive hugs!

Mark Macdonald

Creator of Venice Nutrition

Celebrity Nutritionist

CNN Fitness Expert

New York Times Best Selling Author

PREFACE
Who Are You?

Have you ever looked at yourself in the mirror and wondered, "Who are you?" Not too long ago, I woke up and stumbled to the sink to wash my face. I took off my shirt to get ready for a shower and looked at myself in the mirror. I looked at my reflection and with a puzzled look on my face thought, "Who are you?"

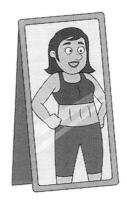
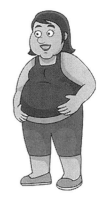

I had let myself go. I was running a successful personal training studio, but I was working from five in the morning until nine at night with an hour commute each way. I had no time to myself, much less to workout, or at least, that was my excuse. I was eating out almost every day and wasn't timing and balancing my meals like I always preached. My marriage was falling apart, and all I could think about was chasing the mighty dollar.

I felt horrible and, more importantly, I was a hypocrite! The funny part is that in my mind, I still had washboard abs. Up until that point, I knew that I had let myself go a little, but it wasn't until my lovely wife made fun of my potbelly that it registered inside my soul that I was getting fat and out of shape.

Here I was working in the health and fitness industry promoting the importance of fitness and helping people lose weight, but I was out of shape and unhealthy. That's when I decided I had to make a change. For all of us, it comes at a different point in our lives. I've seen people in their twenties through their eighties realize that they needed to do something differently in order to lose weight and get healthy.

When people come to meet with a personal trainer, they have usually reached a point where they have tried a number of times to lose weight but have failed. It's also often initiated by some life-altering event. Maybe their doctor told them they needed to start doing something because of potential health risks or maybe they had another big life change, like a divorce or children who were finally old enough so they could start focusing on their health and fitness for a change. In all of these instances, they are ready for a positive change.

The problem is that most people don't know what to do to lose weight or how to get into shape. There is so much misleading information, and it can be very overwhelming to figure out where to start. Lucky for me, I knew what to do, and I had the tools and resources to get back into shape and into the best state of health of my life!

There is a right way and a wrong way to lose weight. I have witnessed so many people losing weight the wrong way, and they typically fall into two categories. The first group is temporarily successful out of sheer willpower. They follow a restrictive diet and starve themselves, or maybe take a fat burner supplement to suppress their appetite.

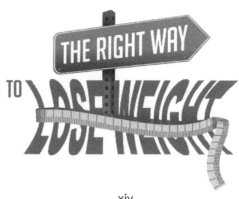

The second group works out but doesn't focus on nutrition. For a long time, I fell into this category. In this group, folks work out for as long as it takes to burn calories and to start seeing results. They will engage in some form of intense cardio or weight training program that ultimately overworks their joints, connective tissues, and muscles to the point of exhaustion or injury.

Unfortunately, these approaches are recipes for disaster. Individuals in both groups always gain the weight back, but it's body fat not the muscle they lost. In fact, they usually gain back more body fat than they had before starting the diet or exercise program in the first place. There is no way to sustain a diet or intense workout routine long term. If you think that diet or exercise alone will help you lose weight, you will fail every time.

This is your wake-up call. I'm here to tell you that there is no diet, magic pill, or specific workout routine that is going to help you lose weight and keep it off for good. I hope you're ready for this. It's going to take hard work. Let me say that again; it's going to take a lot of really freakin' hard work. You are going to have to be dedicated. You are going to have to get used to being uncomfortable. If this is too much for you to handle, then I recommend you stop reading this book. You're not ready to make a change. Until you're sick of being sick and tired, nothing is going to change. For the rest of you, let's get started.

INTRODUCTION
Why It's Not Your Fault

When I started training clients for the first time, I thought I knew how to help them accomplish their fitness goals. I was an athlete and thought that everyone had the discipline and desire to train like they were getting ready for the Olympics. I didn't know a lot about nutrition back then and didn't think it was that important. I thought that as long as you worked out, you could eat whatever you wanted to because that's what I did!

I had never struggled with my weight until the day I looked at myself in the mirror. Yet here I was, trying to help middle-aged women and men lose weight and get healthier. At that time, I had only a few limited life experiences. I didn't understand what it was like to juggle my time so I could care for or spend quality time with a spouse, children, extended family, or friends. I didn't know what it was like to work exhausting hours, meet project deadlines, travel for work meetings, perform church responsibilities, and I'm sure you can fill in the blank with the rest.

I also didn't know what it was like to deal with the self-esteem or emotional and psychological issues that stop us from reaching our goals. I had never tried countless times to lose weight only to fail. To put it mildly, when I first started working with clients, I didn't have a clue what it would take to help them overcome bad habits and learn how to develop a healthy lifestyle. Back then, I would never have been able to help a client lose weight the right way, because I didn't have a system or program to follow. To develop the right program, it took me a couple of years of trial and error while training clients as well as time doing research and consulting with some of the greatest minds in the fitness industry.

Unfortunately, most personal trainers don't know how to help clients in the right way either. Of those individuals who have worked with a personal trainer, less than a quarter say they would work with a personal trainer again. Personal trainers have terrible reputations. In fact, I've had a bad experience with a personal trainer that resulted in a personal vow to never work with one again. Thankfully, I learned from that interaction and was eventually willing to try it again. In fact, that experience was one of the reasons I started in the fitness industry.

Around every corner, there a health club. There are more weight loss, diet, and supplement programs at this moment than in all the past years combined; yet the obesity epidemic is worse than ever before. According to the Centers for Disease Control and Prevention, 75 percent of Americans will be clinically obese by the year 2020. That means that people are going to be so overweight that they will have a hard time doing simple daily tasks, like tying their shoes. How is it that the health and fitness industry is booming, yet we are more obese than we have ever been before?

When I first started working in the fitness industry, I managed a big box gym that was all about production and sales. I want to think that I cared about our clients and gym members, but I was so focused on meeting quotas and revenue targets that I lost sight of what was truly important …you. I would see someone get excited about joining the gym. For the first few weeks, they would come in, but eventually, they would stop working out.

More than 91 percent of people who start an exercise program quit before they ever begin seeing results. 61 percent will give up within the very first week! According to IRHSA (a global community of health and fitness professionals), 67 percent of gym memberships go unused and less than 10 percent of all gym goers work out more than three times in a month.

For people who do use their memberships and go to the gym consistently, very few of them actually see results. I used to watch the same people come into the gym to work out but then never see the weight loss or loss of inches they were hoping for. It was like watching a hamster on a wheel. They would exercise with the best intentions, but they were just going through the same motions and never reaching their goals. If you've been to the gym lately, you've probably seen people do one of three things … cardio, lifting weights, or participating in a class. Unfortunately, they rarely do all three, and they sure don't follow a structured program, track their progress, or have someone holding them accountable to a specific plan.

So, what's the point of all this? I came to the conclusion that the health and fitness industry as a whole was focused on making money and not on improving you and your health. As a personal trainer and health advocate, I knew this wasn't how it should be. I decided I needed to make a change and stand up to what was happening. That's when I started PG FIT. PG FIT stands for Personal and Group Functional Integrated Training. Our mission is to help you accomplish your fitness goals and develop a healthy lifestyle. We have developed a system that will teach you the right way to lose weight.

This book is different from other health and fitness books you may read. This is an instructional book. We are going to teach you a system and program that will help you lose weight the right way so that you can become the healthiest you have been in years. The system is what we call The Five Fundamentals of Health and Fitness. The fundamentals are nutrition, cardio, supplements, resistance training, and coaching. Each fundamental is important to helping you lose weight the right way. You're probably not used to taking notes or writing in a book, but I want you to in this book. I am going to ask you to do a couple of assignments for me. Don't wait until you've read the entire book to go back and complete the assignments. If you can complete them with the right intent, you will get started on a path to losing weight the right way. I promise!

CHAPTER 1

Health vs. Fitness

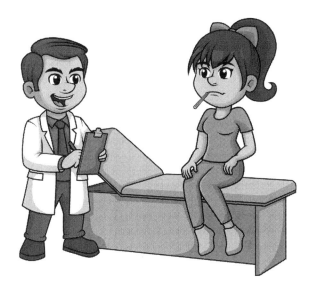

There is a significant distinction between the words "health" and "fitness," but we often use these terms synonymously. People can be healthy but not fit, and people can be fit, but not healthy.

The medical community and insurance companies established health and fitness guidelines in this country. According to the medical community, people are considered "healthy" if they have perfect blood work, pass a physical evaluation with flying colors, and have a normal body mass index (BMI). But does this mean they are physically fit? That's a good question.

Health and fitness standards were established back in the 1950s by insurance companies. The original weight-table standards looked at a person's height-to-weight ratio (or BMI) to determine their overall health. If a person had a high BMI, then they were considered overweight or obese and at a higher risk for developing health-related problems or diseases.

But the tables don't consider a person's body composition or the ratio of their body fat percentage to lean muscle mass. In fact, based on these original weight tables, most world-class bodybuilders or athletes would be categorized as "obese."

This raises an interesting point about the difference between the medical community and health and fitness professionals. Medical professionals typically focus on identifying and treating diseases, while health and fitness professionals work to prevent diseases by encouraging exercise and healthy habits. It's unfortunate that in Western societies, most doctors are trained to start with a pill or surgery rather than looking at your current lifestyle and eating habits to help determine and diagnose any underlying issues that may have caused your disease or illness in the first place.

I learned this firsthand. Some years ago, I developed pain in the upper right quadrant of my abdomen. I had been dealing with the pain for quite some time and had seen many medical professionals about it. They all gave me different opinions about why I had this pain, and it wasn't until I had a gallbladder test that they discovered that my gallbladder was functioning at about 13 percent of its efficiency.

Of course, the surgeon recommended that I have it removed, and I blindly and ignorantly listened to his advice. I have had additional complications since the surgery. Sometimes, the only thing that helps decrease the pain is following a very strict diet with plenty of fruits and vegetables that are high in phytonutrients. Phytonutrients are chemicals or compounds found in plants that have many health benefits. I know others who have had similar interactions with the medical community. A standard or simple procedure doesn't solve a problem, and patients are left with ongoing pain or concerns.

I don't think medical professionals are bad people; rather they just need more information about how to help people with preventative strategies, like diet and exercise. It wasn't until 2010 that medical schools started requiring medical students to take a class on nutrition, and that's only one class in four years of schooling.

Since doctors are supposed to give us advice on how to eat and what we need to do to get into shape, this is a problem. Most of us have followed their counsel, but what we should be doing is evaluating our current lifestyles and diets. Nine times out of ten, these are the culprits. Taking a pill or going under the knife is not always the right solution.

Now, let's consider the other end of the spectrum and consider individuals who are considered incredibly fit, like a bodybuilder or athlete. By all definitions of the word, they are incredibly fit. They have a low body fat percentage, a higher percentage of muscle mass, and can push their bodies to amazing feats. But are they healthy? The average life expectancy of a bodybuilder is right around the young age of 55. It's not because their BMI indicates they are overweight or obese. It is because they have pushed and overworked their bodies and become unhealthy in the process.

I was an athlete and know what it's like to push your body to the extreme. I sacrificed my health to get into the best possible shape for my sport. I would work out too hard and for too long, leading to muscle imbalances, overtraining, and injury. I took too many supplements and drank too many protein shakes because it helped me achieve the results that I was looking for. I was able to compete at a high level, but ultimately, this lifestyle lead to my gallbladder issues and many recurring injuries and issues I have today.

It wasn't until years later that I discovered this anomaly—being healthy does not always lead to fitness, and fitness does not always lead to health. They are not synonymous with each other. You need to work towards achieving balance and moderation on your health and fitness journey. Our goal is to help you become healthy, and then fit. If you just focus on losing weight and neglect your health, then you will miss the point of what we are trying to accomplish. Once you start your journey to becoming healthy, then you can get into the best shape of your life. You have to focus on doing the right things in order to become healthy and fit.

CHAPTER 2
The Five Fundamentals of Health and Fitness

In theory, losing weight should be pretty easy. All you have to do is consume fewer calories than you're burning, and the weight should just fall off. In reality, it isn't that easy or simple. If it were, then everyone would be able to do it.

Losing weight requires a broader approach that focuses on what I like to call The Five Fundamentals of Health and Fitness. The word "fundamental" comes from the Latin word "fundamentum," which means "foundation." The five fundamentals are the foundation for improving your health and fitness. They are the foundation because there is more to losing weight than just moving more and eating less. The five fundamentals consider all aspects of your health and fitness.

If you break down the word "fun-da-mental," you can't deny the fact that your health and fitness journey has to start with emotional and mental preparation before it can start physically. It also has to be a fun and enjoyable process or otherwise you will not be able to sustain your results long term.

The first fundamental is the foundation of your program—nutrition. Approximately 60 to 80 percent of your results come from what you eat. The second fundamental is cardiorespiratory training. This involves a planned and varied approach to improving stamina and heart function. The third fundamental is supplements. These are essential because it's unlikely your diet supplies all the nutrients you need. Supplements can help turbocharge your results. The fourth fundamental is resistance training. This is crucial. Appropriate resistance work (or strength training) strengthens and stabilizes your body while burning calories. The fifth and final fundamental is coaching. You need to work with a coach or fitness professional who will design a program that is motivating and fun, and who will also hold you accountable to it.

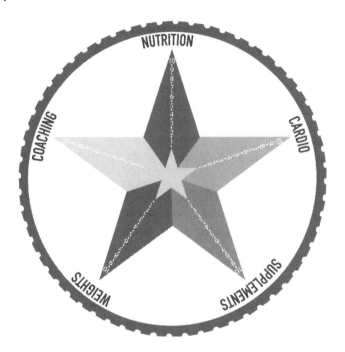

Five Fundamentals Quiz

Imagine the five fundamentals are like the spokes on a bicycle tire. In order to rotate the tire smoothly and effectively, the five elements need to be balanced. To begin, let's determine how balanced you are right now in each category.

Take a moment and read the statements below. If a statement is true for you, then place a checkmark next to it and move to the next one. When you can't answer yes to a statement, circle the number. This shows you where to begin on that particular fundamental.

The first three statements relating to each fundamental help you to identify and recognize certain beliefs and truths you should be aware of and practicing on a daily, weekly, and monthly basis. They help lay down the foundational principles for you to master each fundamental. Statements 4 to 6 help you identify the key behaviors and habits you will need to implement in order to start seeing and achieving results. Statements 7 to 9 help you identify the lifestyle changes you will have to make in order to make the fundamentals a way of life. The last statement for each fundamental is the most important because your success will be dependent on those around you. If you have truly made the fundamentals a way of life, you will also help and empower others to achieve their own health and fitness goals.

Don't worry. When most people start with us, they can't say yes to very many questions (and may not even understand what some of them mean). But our programs are individualized and comprehensive—we go step-by-step and come up with the right plan for you.

Nutrition

1. I understand that 60% to 80% of my results come from nutrition.
2. I drink at least half my body weight in ounces of water daily.
3. I eat five to six small meals daily, especially breakfast.
4. I use my hand as a tool to know portion sizes.
5. I know how many calories I should consume per meal and throughout the day.
6. I balance my macronutrients: protein, fat, and carbs at each meal.

7. I log my food for one week out of each month to review my progress.

8. I periodically weigh and measure my food.

9. I have made my nutrition habits a way of life.

10. I understand the power of blood sugar stabilization and teach it to others—motivating them to make positive changes in their lives.

Aerobic/Cardiorespiratory Training

1. I understand cardio is important for strengthening my heart and lungs and for burning fat.

2. I know both my blood pressure and resting heart rate, and I measure them regularly.

3. I know my target heart rate zones (1 to 5) and use them when training to maximize my results.

4. I do a steady-state, fat-burning cardio workout at least two to three times per week.

5. I have determined my OwnIndex, and my VO2 max is at least 32.

6. I can train in the more advanced target heart rate zones (3 to 4), and I follow an interval program to improve my rate of recovery and fitness.

7. I always use a heart rate monitor when I train and frequently check my progress.

8. I understand the different energy systems, and I can develop a training program to manipulate them.

9. I continuously set cardio goals for myself to improve my cardiorespiratory efficiency and fitness.

10. I understand the importance of cardio training and motivate others to follow a structured cardiovascular program.

Supplements

1. I understand that MOST people do not get the micronutrients they need from their diets.

2. I understand that supplementing my diet can help turbocharge my results, but that I should follow mostly a whole food diet.

3. I know that not all supplements are created equally, and I look for the GMP or USP labels.

4. I take a multivitamin one to two times a day (with food and at intervals throughout the day), or I eat at least 12 to 14 servings of vegetables and fruit daily.

5. I use a high-quality protein powder (hydrolyzed whey or BCAAs) to supplement my protein intake if I don't meet the daily minimum protein requirements.

6. I consume at least three to four servings of calcium-rich foods, or I take at least 1,000 milligrams of calcium daily.

7. I eat at least three to five servings of seafood each week, or I take at least 2,000 milligrams of a high-quality omega complex daily.

8. I periodically take advanced supplements to help cleanse my liver, kidney, and gut or use goal enhancers on an as-needed basis.

9. I eat mostly a whole food diet and supplement it if I am deficient in one or more micronutrients.

10. I share my knowledge about the importance of supplements with others.

Anaerobic/Resistance Training

1. I understand that resistance training is important because it improves my overall health and turns my body into a fat-burning machine.

2. I know that flexibility training is the most important part of a workout.

3. I follow a structured resistance training program two to five times a week.

4. I follow a soft tissue program before working out to break up microscopic tears and adhesions in my muscles.

5. I know exactly what corrective exercises I should be doing to overcome my motor dysfunctions and muscle imbalances.

6. I make sure to incorporate balance, core, and reactive training into every workout.

7. I periodically reassess my biomechanics and perform strength assessments to measure my progress and improve my performance.

8. I know how to properly progress or regress exercises based on my motor dysfunctions or muscle imbalances.

9. I can effectively structure and periodize my own resistance training program.

10. I encourage others to follow a structured resistance training program to improve their overall health.

Coaching

1. I understand that it is important to have a fitness professional to guide me on my health and fitness journey.

2. I have gone through a thorough assessment with a coach. I know my blood pressure and body composition and have gone through a movement screening. I also know what the five fundamentals are.

3. I have defined my "WHY," and I have written down my goals.

4. My coach has explained the importance of nutrition and supplements and has given me nutritional and dietary guidelines to follow.

5. I have had a coach explain the importance of SMFR (self-myofascial release), and I know how to use a foam roller, lacrosse ball, and/or stick to break up muscle tears and adhesions.

6. I have received a structured cardio program, and I know what to do between training days.

7. I know what my motor dysfunctions and band colors are. My coach has effectively explained what correctives exercises I should be doing and which "red light" exercises I should be avoiding.

8. My coach periodically reviews my progress following the five fundamentals (e.g., body comp, biomechanics, fitness testing, etc.).

9. I know I need a coach as an accountability tool. I regularly consult with my coach to review my goals, progress, and program design.

10. My coach is an inspiration to me and serves me to the best of their capabilities.

Based on your responses, how smoothly would your bike tire spin? My guess is your wheel is uneven and probably couldn't make one rotation. Or your wheel is so small that you would have to pedal twice as hard and twice as long to get anywhere. Balancing these fundamentals creates a solid foundation from which you can begin your journey towards health and fitness.

The important part is balance and moderation. When starting a diet or an intense exercise program, you may see results by focusing on just one of the fundamentals, like nutrition or resistance training. But you need to develop an all-encompassing approach if you want to have everlasting results.

Three Ways to Lose Weight

It would seem that losing numbers on the scale would mean you're losing weight. While that's true, it may not be a good thing. There are three different types of weight you can lose—water, muscle, or fat. The last thing that your body wants to lose or burn is body fat. As a defensive and survival mechanism, your body wants to hold on to fat.

When people start to diet or begin an intense exercise program, they generally lose weight within the first few days or weeks. However, they typically lose water and muscle weight because they are not eating or exercising the right way. If you are not fueling your muscles while you are working them, you will start to lose muscle first. Unfortunately, these are the worst types of weight to lose because you're losing the water stored in your muscles and breaking down what lean muscle mass you have. Lean muscle mass is what helps you burn calories. If you start losing your muscle, you're going to burn fewer calories and slow down your metabolic rate.

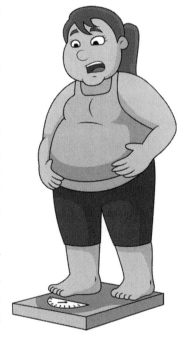

When someone stops a diet or exercise program, what usually happens? They gain the weight back. They don't gain back the muscle they lost. Instead, they only gain fat, and usually more fat than what they started with in the first place. This pattern of losing and gaining weight is called yo-yo dieting. The average person has yo-yo dieted at least three times in their lives, which means that they have lost muscle mass three times and, in the process, gained back more body fat.

The safest and most effective way to lose body fat is to lose it slowly and steadily. The average person can lose about one to two pounds of body fat in a given week. That's important because losing body fat means you're shifting your body composition and gaining muscle, which burns more calories and increases your metabolism.

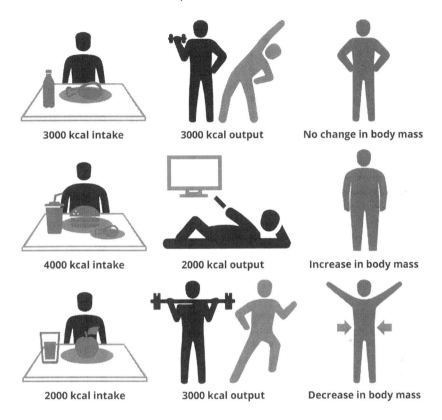

3000 kcal intake	3000 kcal output	No change in body mass
4000 kcal intake	2000 kcal output	Increase in body mass
2000 kcal intake	3000 kcal output	Decrease in body mass

The five fundamentals of health and fitness will help you lose one to two pounds of body fat each week. Nutrition and supplements will account for 60–80 percent of your results by focusing your efforts on how many calories you're taking in by timing and balancing your meals and by taking the right supplements to aid your food intake. Cardiorespiratory and resistance training can help you lose an additional half a pound to a pound of body fat per week. When following structured cardio and resistance training programs, you are able to burn fat efficiently while building the muscle that turns your body into a fat-burning machine. Coaching brings the fundamentals together. A fitness professional can work with you to create a tailored program, help monitor progress, and hold you accountable when you fall off track. There's no need to do it on your own.

Calorie Burn

When trying to lose weight, it's helpful to understand some science. The first law of thermodynamics, the law of conservation of energy, states that the energy that goes into a system has to be equal to or greater than the energy that goes out of the system. In other words, if the number of calories that we consume is greater than what we burn, we will gain weight. Similarly, if it is less than the number of calories we burn, we will lose weight.

There are approximately 3,500 calories in one pound of fat. If you were to create a caloric deficit of 500 calories a day, and you sustained that over seven days, that would equal one pound of weight loss. If it were that simple, though, everybody would be able to lose weight. Unfortunately, it's a little more complicated, and that's why I came up with the five fundamentals.

But let's start by looking at the basics. If you consume 3,000 calories and you only burn 2,000 calories, there is a 1,000 calorie surplus. You will gain weight, most likely body fat. If you consume 2,000 calories and you burn 3,000 calories, there is a 1,000 calorie deficit. If that is sustained over seven days (1,000 calories x 7 days a week = 7,000 calories) that equals a weight loss of two pounds.

If you consume 2,000 calories and you burn 2,000 calories, then it's even. There's not necessarily going to be a change in your body mass. When you attain a weight loss or body fat percentage goal, you then want to balance your caloric intake so it matches the energy you use. Achieving your goal is where the magic happens because you will be able to consume as many calories as you're burning and still be able to maintain your results.

Now let's say that somebody didn't change anything about their diet and decided to lose weight by only exercising. That sounds like a pretty simple solution, right? You would have to burn an extra 500 calories a day and sustain that for seven days to lose one pound of fat. The average person burns approximately 100 calories for every mile that they run. To lose one pound of fat just with exercise, you would have to run approximately five miles a day to burn that extra 500 calories, and you'd have to do that seven days a week. That's 35 miles of running throughout the week to burn 3,500 calories. Does that seem so simple now?

You also have to consider that after about three to four weeks of following this intense running program, your body would physiologically adapt. It would figure out how to do the same amount of work while burning fewer calories. As you get more fit (whether it's running or something else), you will start to burn approximately half as many calories as you did when you initially started. What that means is you'll need to run twice as far just to lose the same amount of weight. You'd have to run upwards of 70 miles in a week to burn 3,500 calories to lose one pound of fat.

These are just a few examples of why losing weight isn't as straightforward as it seems it should be. It's also why I work with my clients to structure a program tailored to their individual needs and based on the five fundamentals. Coaching, combined with a comprehensive approach that targets nutrition, cardiorespiratory training, supplements, and resistance training, makes the difference.

CHAPTER 3
Are Your Goals SMART?

If you aim at nothing, you will hit it every time.

–Zig Ziglar

Each of us probably understands the importance of setting goals, whether for work or health. But sometimes determining what goals to set can be challenging. I frequently encounter this with clients who aren't quite sure where to begin, especially if they have failed before. This may make them want to give up on themselves and their health and fitness. Luckily, they have a coach who will work with them to move forward.

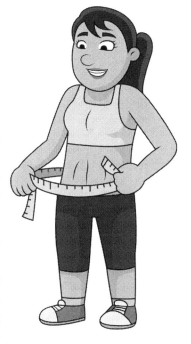

Even with a coach, identifying and setting goals is only successful if you prioritize attaining them. Many people are successful in other areas of their lives, but health and fitness take a back seat to other responsibilities. Their job or kids come first, while health and fitness have typically been their last priority. To reach your goals, be ready to work for them and for yourself.

What are your health and fitness goals? What do you want to accomplish? If you're reading this book, one of your goals might be to lose weight. But I want you to think bigger. Losing weight cannot be the most important goal. Your goal should answer the questions, "Why do I want to lose weight?" and "Why is it important?" Identifying and understanding your "why" is going to be the driving force that helps you stay motivated to reach your health and fitness goal.

How to Set Goals

I recently met with a client, Kathy, who wanted to lose 20 to 30 pounds to get back to her senior year of college weight. Her husband worked all the time, and her kids were in high school, so it was time for her to start focusing on herself instead of her husband and kids.

I love a great weight loss story, so we got started. At PG Fit, the goalsetting process begins by talking about general goals and then getting baseline numbers for body weight and body composition. After analyzing Kathy's body composition numbers, we found that she needed to lose closer to 35 pounds of fat mass, not just the 20 to 30 pounds she had mentioned. She had yo-yo dieted for so many years that she had lost a lot of her muscle. Now, she needed to lose body fat and gain muscle to reach her goal.

I proceeded to ask her my second, but more important, question, "Why do you want to lose 35 pounds of fat?" She looked at me a little puzzled because she had never really thought about why she wanted to get back to her college weight. She knew that she needed to lose weight, but she had not questioned her motivation.

I explained that to reach her goal, she would need a more powerful reason than numbers on a scale. She needed to find a purpose that would get her up in the morning and to the gym, even when she may not feel like going to the gym that day. This driving force was going to motivate her to log her food and avoid the glasses of wine with her girlfriends on Thursday nights.

When she thought about it for a second, she said she was turning 50 this year, and she was planning a big birthday celebration with her family and friends. I thought to myself, "Okay, now we're getting somewhere." I asked her why it was important to look good at her fiftieth birthday party. She thought about it for several minutes, and with tears forming in her eyes, she broke down and told me that the year her mother had turned 50, she had a stroke.

She told me how devastating it was to see her mother's health decline and that her mother was never the same after the stroke. She also talked about the undue stress and burden that it put on her family, something she never wanted her husband or kids to have to go through. Bingo! We had found her "why"! I told her that when she feels like giving up or that it's too hard to lose the weight, she needs to think about her mother, but more importantly, she needs to think about her husband and two kids who need her to be there for them.

Our "why" has to be so powerful that it makes us emotional just to think about it. Now, I want you to write out your goals. You can't just have them in your head. Statistically speaking, you are 80 percent more likely to reach your goals if they are written down.

What are my health and fitness goals? Be very specific!

_____

_____

_____

_____

_____

Why are these goals important to you? My "why" is…

_____

_____

_____

_____

_____

SMART Goals

Once you've determined why you want to attain a specific goal, it's time to strategize and plan so you can achieve that goal. At PG Fit, we work with clients to be sure their goals are SMART. SMART is an acronym that stands for—Specific, Measurable, Attainable, Relevant, and Time-bound.

Your goal to lose weight has to be SMART. You can't just set a goal to lose weight; you need a plan and structure. Let's look at an example of the SMART planning process.

Specific

You've decided you want to lose weight. A SMART-based plan would make that goal more specific. For instance, I want to lose 35 pounds of body fat, or I want to get my body fat percentage down to 25 percent.

Measurable

The second step is to make sure that you can track and measure your results along the way. Maybe you commit to a weekly weigh-in at your gym, where they have a bioelectrical impedance scale that measures your body fat. Remember you can't just focus on weight loss because there are three different types of weight loss, and you want to make sure that you're focusing primarily on losing body fat.

Attainable

The next step is to make sure that your goal is attainable. This is going to be different for everyone and will be dependent on your current behaviors, habits, and lifestyle choices.

Trying to lose 20 pounds in a month is probably not attainable, especially if you are used to eating fast food every day. But, if you're following the five fundamentals of health and fitness, the average person can lose one to two pounds of body fat mass per week. The average person could lose 35 pounds of body fat in 18 to 35 weeks.

Relevant

This step is a lot like your "why." It makes sure that your goal is relevant and in alignment with what's important to you, your family, and your priorities. It has to be your goal and not something someone else thinks you should work towards, for example, your spouse. In Kathy's case, it was important to stay healthy for her family. It has to be relevant so that you will stay motivated even when it gets hard.

Time

And the final step is to make sure that your goal has start and finish dates. You have to set a specific date for when you want to accomplish your goal. Sometimes that's before a big event or trip. Other times, it's just the end of 30 days. Whatever you choose, stick to it.

Goal Card

Use PG Fit's SMART Goal card to help you set your health and fitness goals. Remember, writing down your health and fitness goals and creating an action plan makes it far more likely you will accomplish them.

We have organized the goal card into three commitments. First, write down specifically what your goal is. I want to ... (something like) "lose 35 pounds of body fat."

Second, set a date for when you want to reach your goal. Write down the exact day, whether it's 35 weeks or nine months from today.

Finally, write out specifically what you will do to achieve your goal—at least three things that you can focus on.

These specific actions will help you reach your goal. They may be something you're currently not doing at all or just something that you need to improve. Three actions might include: I will log food daily and keep track of how many calories I'm taking in. Or, I will reduce my alcohol intake to one to three glasses of wine per week. Or, lastly, I will go to the gym four times a week and follow a structured cardio program for two days a week.

Once you have filled out the My SMART Goal card, you are well on your way to reaching your goal. I am so proud of you for making it this far. Next, we're going to be talking specifically about each of the five fundamentals and how they can help you accomplish your health and fitness goals.

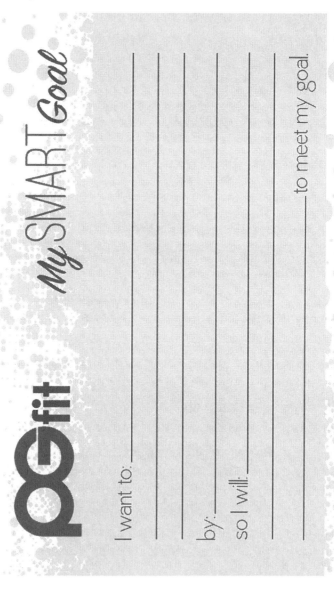

CHAPTER 4

You Can't Out Train a Bad Diet

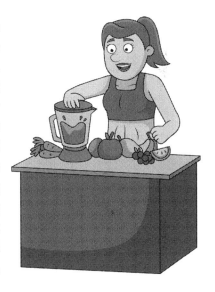

Nutrition is the first of the five fundamentals because it is the foundation of the entire structure. What you eat becomes the fuel that drives all other aspects of your training. Approximately 60 to 80 percent of your results are based on what you eat. I've found that it's also one of the most challenging components for many clients. Starting and maintaining a healthy diet that supports weight management and a healthy lifestyle takes thought, planning, and persistence.

Additionally, what we eat is very personal. It's influenced by our upbringing, experiences, and habits. We all have different belief systems based on how we were raised and what we have been conditioned to do. These factors result in each of us having different philosophies and approaches to nutrition that can be tough to shift.

When I was a child, it was feast or famine. I am the oldest of five children. When my parents returned from the grocery store, my siblings and I would rush the pantry to devour and hide our favorite snacks. It was a blood sport event in our household to see who could get the Ding Dongs and the Little Debbie Star Crunches. If you've never had a Star Crunch, imagine a chocolate-covered rice crispy treat with all the artificial flavors and preservatives you can think of. It was heaven in your mouth.

It wasn't until years later that I realized that eating two or three Star Crunches wasn't what they meant by carb-loading before a competition. I also didn't know until years later that I suffered from empty-plate syndrome. A nutritionist explained to me that I didn't have to eat everything on my plate and that I should stop eating when I was satiated or full. While this made perfect sense, it was a tricky one for me to follow. It was a rule in our house that you couldn't leave the table until you had eaten everything on your plate. I'm sure that you went through some experiences like these as well!

Diet vs. Nutrition

When you hear the word diet, what do you think of? I think of all the popular diets out there, like Atkins, Jenny Craig, Weight Watchers, the Paleo diet, and the Ketogenic diet. Guess what? All diets are successful temporarily. It doesn't matter which diet you follow; you will see temporary results. All diets reduce your caloric intake and manipulate your macronutrient percentages. Your macronutrients are protein, fat, and carbohydrates. You will always lose weight if you are taking in fewer calories than you are burning.

What do the first three letters of the word diet spell? D. I. E. All diets are successful temporarily, but in the end, they fail. The word diet, by definition, simply means the food we consume. But since the 1970s, when some of the first diets started becoming mainstream in America, we have misused and abused the word diet. You shouldn't adhere to or follow any limiting or restrictive diet.

Additionally, many diets result in losing the wrong type of weight. Remember the three different types of weight loss? You can lose fat, water, or muscle. You want to lose fat, but restrictive diets or decreasing carbohydrate intake may result in weight loss that is primarily water and muscle.

Instead, we need to think about what we eat from a nutritional perspective, which means there are several important concepts to understand. These concepts do not include our philosophy or beliefs. They are basic laws of science. The first we've already mentioned— the first law of thermodynamics, also known as law of conservation of energy. It states that the relationship between the calories we consume and the calories we burn impacts whether we gain or lose weight.

Not All Calories Are Created Equal

However, not all calories are equal. Think of it this way. Eating 1,000 calories of Star Crunches (or fat) will have a completely different physiological effect on your body than eating 1,000 calories of chicken (or lean protein). How your body breaks down fat and protein is based on a principle known as the specific dynamic action of food.

Essentially, your body has to work harder to break down and metabolize protein versus carbohydrates or fat. This is important because your body will burn more calories breaking down protein than the other macronutrients. In fact, your body will have to work about ten times harder to break down proteins versus fats and almost five times harder to break down proteins versus carbohydrates. Fats don't require much work for your body to use them as an energy source or to store for energy use later on. This is where an awareness of nutrition comes into play. We have to understand the elements of healthy eating in order to eat well and optimize our performance.

I used to think that I could eat whatever I wanted as long as I trained hard. When I was younger, I could get away with it and never gain weight, but that was because I was working out several hours a day. I was burning just as many calories as I was taking in, and I needed many of those empty calories. It wasn't until years later that I started to view food as fuel and became more conscious of what I ate.

An important part of viewing food as fuel involves understanding how the body processes this fuel. Different foods generate different types of energy, and how your body burns that energy impacts your performance. Imagine your body is like a car. We'll equate your metabolism (or how quickly you burn calories) to a car's miles per gallon. A small Toyota Prius is going to get better gas mileage than a big pickup truck or eighteen-wheeler. Similarly, we all have different body types, so we are all going to have different metabolic rates (or miles per gallon). A tall, muscular person is going to have a higher metabolism (or get more miles per gallon) than a smaller, less muscular person.

Over time, as a car or your body begins to age, your metabolism or miles per gallon will slow down as well. While genetics plays a role in body type and metabolism, you control your nutrition and activity. Once you start to understand that food is fuel and the type of fuel you provide your body affects how you burn energy, you will begin to make better food choices. Choosing balanced foods that power your body and timing your meals throughout the day will have an enormous impact on your health and fitness. Essentially, you are what you eat!

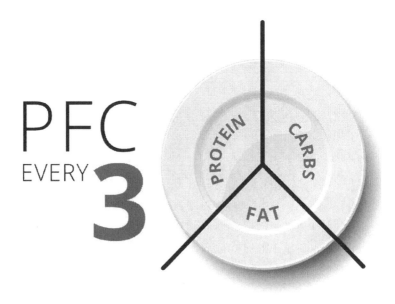

PFC
EVERY 3
PROTEIN CARBS FAT

Macronutrients

Once you have a big-picture understanding of nutrition, it's time to look at the importance of balancing your macronutrients—proteins, fats, and carbohydrates. A macronutrient is basically something that is vital or essential for life. At PG Fit, we call these your PFCs, which stands for proteins, fats, and carbohydrates. I want you to think of them in that specific order and be sure to consume these three macronutrients at every meal.

At each meal, you want to think—Where is my protein? Where is my fat? Where is my carbohydrate? Your diet is going to consist of about 10–40 percent protein, 20–30 percent fat, and 40–70 percent carbohydrates. These ratios are going to be slightly different for each person because of body type and metabolism.

Imagine your metabolism is like a fire, and the goal is to keep the fire burning all day long. Your macronutrients are the three things the fire needs to keep burning. I like to compare them to wood, coal, and gasoline. Protein is the wood, maintaining a steadily burning fire. Fat acts like the coals, providing a long burning fire. Carbohydrates are like gasoline and get the fire going quickly (and also burn out faster).

At each meal, you want to have each element represented in the right proportion so you can fuel your body. You want to repeat this process every three to four hours. That's the "every three" in PFC Every 3! Think of a baby. How often does a baby eat? A baby eats every few hours. Breast milk or formula is a perfect balance of protein, fat, and carbohydrates, and that is the way we should be eating. As human beings, we should be eating every three to four hours to maintain our energy levels, avoid hunger, and more importantly, fuel our bodies the right way. It's not rocket science. If a baby knows how to eat at birth, maybe we are just overcomplicating, and letting society dictate when we should be eating!

Protein

Amino acids are the building blocks of proteins, and they are essential for your body to build and repair cells. Proteins are also needed for tissue synthesis and the regulation of specific bodily functions. There are two different types of proteins—complete and incomplete. Generally speaking, animal proteins are complete, and plant proteins are incomplete.

When you consume protein, complete proteins are important. I tell people to think of the mother concept. At each meal, you should include foods that came from a mother. That means things like beef, chicken, turkey, fish, eggs, dairy products, etc. Incomplete sources of protein include beans, nuts, seeds, etc. Everyone's diet is a little different, but you should strive to eat complete proteins at least three times a day or a variety of incomplete sources to ensure adequate protein intake.

Fat

Fats (or lipids) are comprised of fatty acids, which form phospholipids or triglycerides. Phospholipids and triglycerides are other forms of fat. Your body uses fats as fuel. In fact, you need to eat fat to burn body fat.

Fats are typically broken down into two categories—saturated and unsaturated. Saturated fats (generally animal fats) are solid at room temperature, while unsaturated fats (generally plant fats) are typically liquid at room temperature. Fats are essential for flavor and digestion. They also provide our bodies with essential fatty acids. Some examples of fats include oils, nut butters, avocadoes, as well as the "invisible fats" that are found in meats, poultry, fish, and dairy products. Even if you think you are eating a lean piece of meat, there is fat marbled in the meat, making it a source of "invisible fats."

Carbohydrates

Carbohydrates support all of our vital functions, and we could not live without them. The building blocks for carbohydrates are sugars called monosaccharides, disaccharides, and polysaccharides. Carbohydrates can be categorized as complex or simple.

Complex carbohydrates are harder to break down than simple carbohydrates. Eventually, both complex and simple carbohydrates are broken down into glucose or converted to glycogen, which is our body's primary source for fuel. However, if you eat too many carbohydrates, they can easily be converted to fat.

Some examples of complex carbohydrates include brown rice, oatmeal, pasta, potatoes, quinoa, vegetables, and fruit. Some examples of simple carbohydrates are honey, maple syrup, and sugar. At the end of the day, sugar is sugar, and it doesn't matter if it comes from complex or simple carbohydrates.

As I mentioned above, we can't live without carbohydrates. Without them, we would die. You also cannot metabolize fat without carbohydrates. Carbohydrates are our body's primary source for fuel and support all of our vital functions. Eating the right kind of carbohydrates will help you lose weight and burn fat efficiently. They will fill you up, curb your hunger, control your blood sugar to help you burn fat, speed up your metabolism, and keep you satisfied and feeling good.

Portions

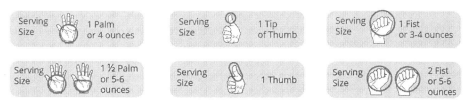

Even if you eat all the right foods, you can still gain weight if you don't pay attention to portion size. The easiest way to measure portion sizes is to use your hand as a guide.

For women, a serving of protein should be three to four ounces, which is about the size of your palm. For men, a serving is typically five to six ounces, which is one and a half to two palms.

For fats, a serving size is much smaller. For women, that means anywhere from one to two ounces, which is approximately the tip of your thumb. For men, a serving ranges from three to five ounces, or your whole thumb.

The serving size for carbohydrate portions can also be measured using your hand. For women, a serving size of three to four ounces should be about one fist. For men, a serving of five to six ounces is more like two fists.

If you use your hand as a way to measure your portion sizes and you're eating a balance of protein, fat, and carbohydrates at least every three to four hours, you're almost certainly going to start losing weight the right way.

Blood Sugar Stabilization

Another important principle to understand is the power of blood sugar stabilization. Your body wants to maintain homeostasis, or balance. Ideally, your blood sugar should be somewhere between 80 and 120 milligrams per deciliter.

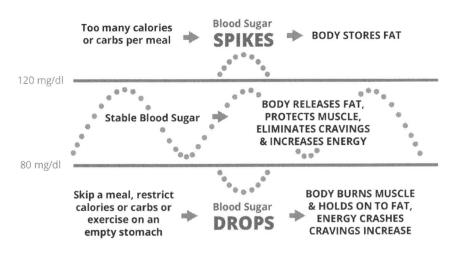

When you start consuming too many calories or carbohydrates, your blood sugar (glucose levels) can spike above 120 milligrams per deciliter. When this happens, you start storing body fat. At the same time, insulin is released by the pancreas to bring your blood sugar levels back down, and this causes blood sugar to be stored in your fat cells.

When you skip a meal (especially breakfast) or if you go longer than three to four hours without eating, your blood sugar levels can also drop below 80 milligrams per deciliter, and you start burning muscle. The pancreas counters this by releasing glucagon, which gets the liver to release glucose or blood sugar back into the blood to restore your blood sugar levels. This is known as glycogenolysis.

If blood sugar levels are too low, your body will pull the glucose or blood sugar from your muscles in a process known as gluconeogenesis. The goal is to keep your blood sugar between 80 and 120 milligrams per deciliter to make sure that you're primarily burning fat.

Ideally, blood sugar levels remain stable, so fat is released into the bloodstream. It's then absorbed by the muscles and used as energy. Fat is primarily burned in your muscles. If you're not eating every three to four hours and balancing your protein, fat, and carbohydrates (PFCs) at each meal, there is no way that you can efficiently burn body fat.

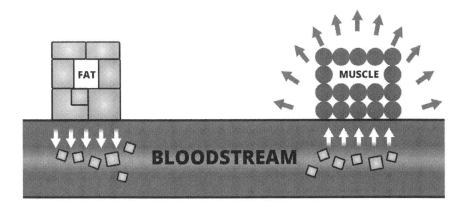

To keep blood sugar levels balanced, it's important to try and eat every three to four hours. While this can be difficult to do because we're often on the go, it is essential if you are trying to balance your PFCs. The best way to be successful managing the PFC Every 3 Rule is to prepare and plan a couple of meals in advance. Keeping PFCs balanced by eating every three to four hours is essential. Otherwise, the benefits are lost because you'll eat, spike your blood sugar levels, and then store the fat.

Eat Smart Summary

1. Drink at least 16 to 32 ounces of water and eat within 30 to 60 minutes after waking up. This will hydrate your body and jump-start your metabolism. You have all heard the saying that breakfast is the most important meal of the day. It's true!

2. Eat every three to four hours, which means five to six smaller meals throughout the day. This speeds up your metabolic rate and minimizes hunger cravings, which can lead to binge eating later in the day or at night.

3. Eat a balance of protein, fat, and carbohydrates at each meal. Use your hand as a guide to measure your portion sizes. Each meal should consist of lean proteins, healthy fats, and complex carbohydrates, which should mostly come from fruits and vegetables.

4. Prepare and plan your meals in advance. I can't emphasize enough the importance of making sure that you spend at least a couple of hours each week preparing and planning your meals in advance.

The easiest way to incorporate these rules into your life is to focus on adding one new rule each week. Focus on that one item and make it work. In this way, you are always working towards success.

Meal Plans

I have also provided a simple meal plan to follow below. Hundreds of PG Fit clients have used this one meal plan to learn how to eat the right way. You can follow the plan precisely as it is designed, or you can substitute some of the foods for other choices you might like better. On the first page, I provide an overview of each meal with different food options.

PGfit

TIME	FOODS	NOTES
BREAKFAST	Omelet or Meal Replacement Shake MEAL REPLACEMENT OPTIONS INCLUDE CORE Shake, Proto Whey w/Fruit, ETC.	CAN DRINK SHAKE WITH 1/2 CUP OF MILK (DAIRY, SOY OR ALMOND) OPTIMALLY, USE ONLY WATER
MID MORNING	Meal Replacement Bar OPTIONS INCLUDE: Power Crunch Bar Advanced Athletics Bar, Quest, Think Thin, etc.	CAN HAVE A QUICK MEAL INSTEAD, LIKE TURKEY SLICES W/NUTS & FRUIT OR STRING CHEESE & FRUIT
LUNCH	Your Meal Choice	CHOOSE MEAL FROM YOUR FOOD PLAN. EX: SANDWICH/WRAP OR PROTEIN PACKED SALAD
MID AFTERNOON	Meal Replacement Shake OPTIONS INCLUDE: Proto Whey w/Fruit, CORE Shake, etc.	CAN DRINK SHAKE WITH 1/2 CUP OF MILK (DAIRY, SOY OR ALMOND) OPTIMALLY, USE ONLY WATER
DINNER	Your Meal Choice	CHOOSE MEAL FROM YOUR FOOD PLAN. EX: SALMON W/ BROWN RICE & ASPARAGUS OR PROTEIN PACKED STIR FRY
NIGHTTIME (DEPENDS ON SCHEDULE)	Your Meal Choice	CHOOSE MEAL FROM YOUR FOOD PLAN. EX: GREEK YOGURT W/ ALMONDS & BLUEBERRIES OR HARD-BOILED EGG & RASPBERRIES

You should make sure you're eating the following meals: breakfast, midmorning snack, lunch, midafternoon snack, dinner, and occasionally a nighttime meal. Remember, you should also be eating every three to four hours and balance your protein, fat, and carbohydrates at each meal.

The next chart provides detailed information to help you understand how to measure your intake of protein, fats, and carbohydrates. It also gives examples in each category. If you are going to drink alcohol, we recommend replacing your carb with a glass of alcohol. The bottom of the chart shows free foods or spices and condiments you can use to cook with to add flavor and enhance the taste of your macronutrients.

FOOD PLAN FOR FEMALES

Protein (choose 1 per meal)
(20-25 grams per meal)

Fats (choose 1 per meal)
(7-8 grams per meal)

Carbs (choose 1 per meal)
(20 grams per meal)

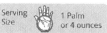 Serving Size — 1 Palm or 4 ounces

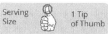 Serving Size — 1 Tip of Thumb

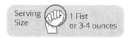 Serving Size — 1 Fist or 3-4 ounces

Lean:
- Chicken
- Cottage Cheese
- Egg Whites
- Fish (lean)
- Greek Yogurt
- Hemp Powder
- Hydrolyzed Whey (i.e proto whey)
- Tofu
- Turkey Breast
- (all fresh /frozen meat)

Non Lean:
(do not choose fat w/ this option)
- Eggs Whole
- Beef (filet)
- Beef (ground 99% lean)
- Fish (non-lean)
- Lamb
- Pork

- Avocado
  (1.5 oz, about ¼ of an avocado)
- Butter (½ tablespoon)
- Flaxseed Oil (½ tablespoon)
- Mayo (1.5 tablespoon low fat)
- Nut Butter (1 tablespoon)
- Nuts (.5 oz, about 12)
- Olive Oil (½ tablespoon)
- Salad Dressing (1 tablespoon)
- Sour Cream (1 tablespoon)

We suggest measuring your foods for 7 days to optimize your results.

Recommended Supplements
- Liquid Antioxidants (4oz / day)
- Omega 3 (3000-5000mg / day)

Fruit:
- Apples
- Banana
- Berries
- Mango
- Orange
- (all fruits)

Vegetables:
- Broccoli
- Cucumber
- Eggplant
- Green Beans
- Onions
- Spinach
- Tomato
- (all veggies)

Grains / Calorie Dense Carbs:
- Beans (½ cup ckd)
- Bread / Wrap (less than 80 cals)
- Brown Rice (½ cup ckd)
- Oatmeal / Hot Cereals (.75 oz)
- Pasta (fist sized)
- Potatoes (3 oz)
- Quinoa (½ Cup ckd)

Alcohol (replace carbs in meal with alcohol)
Wine (6oz) | Liquor (1 shot) | Beer (12 oz)
(Limit to 1 serving 1-2 times/week)
Alcohol is optional

Free Foods
- All Seasonings / Spices
  (including salt & pepper)
- Citrus Juice or Zest (lemon/lime)
- Fat Free Cooking Spray (like Pam)
- Capers
- Extracts (vanilla, almond, etc.)
- Garlic & Shallots

- Horseradish
- Mustard + Ketchup (low sugar)
- Lettuce, Tomato, Onion
  (sandwich qty.)
- Sriracha Sauce
- Stevia (natural sweetener)
- Vinegar (balsamic, red wine, etc.)
- Worcestershire Sauce

Water
- 2-3 liters per day
  (8-12 glasses)
  (the more the better)

Take your body weight and multiply it by 66% to figure out exactly how much water to drink.

It's also important to make sure you are drinking enough water every day. The best way to determine how much water you should be drinking is to take your body weight and multiply it by 66 percent to figure out exactly how many ounces of water you should be drinking.

The final chart reviews food quality ranging from least processed to most processed. Within these categories, each macronutrient is

QUALITY OF FOOD CHART

Highest Quality:
Least Processed and Least Refined

Protein	Carbohydrates	Fats
• Beef	• Beans - Fresh	• Avocado
• Chicken	• Brown Rice	• Flaxseed Oil
• Egg Whites	• Fruit	• Natural Nut Butter
• Egg Whole	• Hot Cereals	• Nuts
• Fish	• Sweet Potatoes	• Olive Oil
• Hemp Powder	• Vegetables	• Olives
• Hydrolyzed Whey (i.e proto whey)	• Yams	
• Pork		
• Turkey Breast		
• Whey Protein - Grass-Fed		
(all other fresh / frozen meat)		

Medium Quality:
Medium Processed and Medium Refined

Protein	Carbohydrates	Fats
• Canned Meat	• Bread	• Canola Oil
• Garden Burgers	(at least 2 grams of fiber)	• Guacamole
• Pre-Packaged Meats	• Canned Beans	• Processed Nut
• Protein Powder - Whey, Egg & Soy	• Canned Fruit	Butters
• Sandwich Meats	• Canned Vegetables	• Vegetable Oil
• Soy Beans	• Cold Cereals	
• Soy Meat - Packaged	• Crackers	
• Quorn	• Pasta	
• Dairy	• Potatoes, Red & White	
- Cheese	• Pretzels	
- Cottage Cheese		

Low Quality:
Most Processed and Most Refined

Protein	Carbohydrates	Fats
• Protein Bars (non-hydrolyzed)	• Bread	• Butter
• RTD Protein (non-hydrolyzed)	(< 2 grams of fiber)	• Creamy Salad
(ready to drink)	• Ice Cream	Dressing
	• Potato Chips	• Margarine
	• Tortilla Chips	• Mayonaise
	• White Rice	• Sour Cream

broken down into high-, medium-, and low-quality foods. The goal is to eat foods that are the least processed. Ideally, you should be having at least three high-quality meals throughout the day as well as a couple of snacks. We recommend using high-quality meal replacement shakes or protein bars, but you can also have one to two medium- or low-quality meals, using the guidelines below. Be careful because the low-quality foods are the most processed and refined, and they will spike your blood sugar!

If you're feeling a little overwhelmed, don't worry. Most people don't know where to begin when it comes to picking out good foods. Basically, just try to eat as many natural things as you possibly can. If something has more than five ingredients or several ingredients you don't know how to pronounce, you should think twice about buying it! Also, picking fat-free or sugar-free foods is the wrong way to go. These foods are loaded with artificial or genetically modified ingredients. Don't fall for food manufacturers' marketing gimmicks. If something seems to be too good to be true, then it probably is!

It also doesn't have to cost a fortune to eat right. Not everyone can eat all organic or fresh foods from the local farmer's market. Just try to do your best to pick healthy options!

Food Log

The last concept we want to talk about is the importance of logging your food and counting your calories. This is especially important when starting out, so you have an accurate understanding of how many calories you're 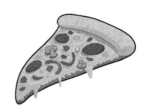 eating and how many you're burning. Most people underestimate their caloric consumption by about 48 percent. That means that most people think they are eating 2,000 calories a day when they are eating closer to 3,000 calories a day.

How many calories do you think are in an average slice of pepperoni pizza? Most people would guess 200 or maybe 250 calories. If you take the median of some of the most popular pizza joints, there are approximately 500 calories in a slice of pepperoni pizza. Do you find that surprising? I challenge you to look up some of your favorite foods. I bet you would be surprised!

You will have to log your food for a minimum of seven days if you want to honestly know how many calories you are taking in and what your macronutrient balance looks like. I would recommend logging your food for seven days without changing anything about your diet so that you can see what your diet looks like. I can promise you that it will be an eye-opening experience (as it is for me every time I do it). You can do anything for seven days!

Thanks to technology, there are many easy ways to log your food. Most of our clients rely on apps that make it easy to keep track of your food intake. Popular ones include MyFitnessPal, dotFIT, and Lose It!. At one point, we even created a PG Fit app so that our clients could log their food. If you want to understand the importance of nutrition and how to log your food, you should make sure to write it down. There's something magical about writing down your food instead of just logging it into an app.

You can use an app to help you collect the information, but when you physically write down what you're consuming, how many calories are in each food, and what the macronutrient breakdown looks like, it helps you consciously understand how much food you're actually consuming. It helps you start to think twice about eating certain foods, and you will begin to make better food choices and develop better habits!

At some point, you're going to have to track what you're eating. But if you're not ready to take that quantum leap, you can get started by using your hand as a guide to measure your portion sizes. You will still see some great results!

The Weekend

Like most of our clients, you will probably do well Monday through Thursday when you're on a schedule and it's easy to stay pretty disciplined. During the week, logging food and tracking progress is part of a regular day. You may even be able to create a caloric deficit of about 500 to 1,000 calories a day. That's pretty good and would give you at least a 2,000 calorie deficit for the week. But then, the weekend happens.

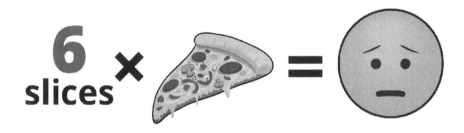

On Friday night, people like to go out to dinner or order take out. Whatever your vice is, maybe it's a glass of wine, chips and salsa, or a couple of beers, let's imagine you get together with friends for a pizza party. Maybe you have six slices of pizza. Well, if the average slice contains about 500 calories and you have six slices, that's the equivalent of taking in an additional 3,000 calories. If you created a 2,000 calorie deficit Monday through Thursday, but you consume 3,000 in one meal, then you have just negated all the hard work you did throughout the week, and that's only one meal.

Now, just imagine what happens on Saturday and Sunday. People typically don't eat very well all weekend, and a lot of time we aren't as active as we are during the week, especially on Sundays. One day can set you back all week, and one weekend can set you back a few weeks. That's why it's critical to keep track of your food every single day for seven days. You know what you're eating. Even if you only start by writing down foods (and don't track calories or macronutrients), you'll have a great beginning and a lot of useful information. I know you can do it!

When I first started training, I didn't understand the importance of nutrition. I worked out a lot and figured that meant I could eat whatever I wanted, but that was completely wrong. For optimal health and performance, you need to eat well. You can't out train a bad diet. In fact, about 60 to 80 percent of your results are based on what you're eating. When you understand that fueling your body is based on science rather than the latest fad diet, you discover the power of eating the right way!

CHAPTER 5

How to Stop Spinning Your Wheels

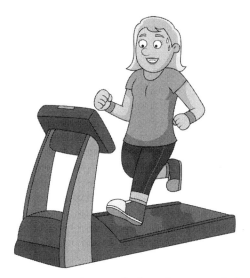

Cardiorespiratory training (or cardio) is the second fundamental. The reason that cardio is the second fundamental is that the heart is the most important muscle group in the human body. Your heart is like an engine in a car. Without it, you would not be able to power your body. It's important to strengthen your heart and lungs to provide your body and working muscles with the blood, nutrients, and oxygen they need to function efficiently. Besides nutrition, cardio is extremely important to improving your overall health and fitness.

If you have been to the gym lately, you have probably seen people who are on the cardio equipment for a long time; but you may question, are they working out efficiently? When I worked at the big-box gym, I would see people spend countless hours running on a treadmill, using the elliptical, or riding a stationary bike. I would see them sweating and working hard, but I would never see their body composition change over time.

It reminded me of when I was a little kid, and my younger brother got a pet gerbil. The gerbil would get on the comfort wheel and start running. I thought it was the funniest thing. The gerbil would run and run, and the wheel would spin and spin, but the gerbil would never get anywhere.

Similarly, if you're not following a structured cardio program, you are just like a gerbil on a wheel. You're spinning your wheels, and you will not see results. The goal with cardio training is to learn how to maximize your results in the shortest amount of time. When you follow a structured cardio program, you will know what your target heart rate should be and know the amount of time you need to keep it there in order to strengthen your heart and lungs and burn fat.

Healthy Heart

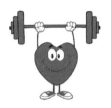

There are two primary systems that are improved by cardiorespiratory training—cardiovascular and pulmonary. Your cardiovascular system consists of your heart, blood, and blood vessels. What makes a car move? The engine! What's the most important muscle group in your body? Your heart! If your heart and cardiovascular system aren't working efficiently, you are in big trouble. Your pulmonary system includes your lungs, bronchioles, etc. It delivers oxygen throughout your body. If you're unable to supply oxygen throughout your body efficiently, you're also in big trouble.

So what happens when you work your heart by doing cardio activities? Well, it's pretty simple. As you train and improve your cardio capabilities, your cardiovascular and respiratory systems become more efficient. Cardio leads to an increase in the size and strength of your heart, which makes you stronger and healthier.

When you first start a cardio program, your respiratory system may struggle to provide sufficient amounts of oxygen to the different parts of your body. At this point, your body needs to develop the ability to pump more blood to accommodate the greater volume of blood demanded by working muscles. To do this, your heart will need to increase in size and strength to push more blood and oxygen throughout your body.

Cardiorespiratory training, also called aerobic training, works the heart to make it stronger. Aerobic effort requires oxygen to produce energy. In contrast, resistance training is called anaerobic training. Anaerobic implies that oxygen is not needed to produce energy. We'll talk more about anaerobic training later. In both instances, your body wants to burn sugar or carbohydrates as a fuel. It then breaks down this fuel into a usable form of energy called adenosine triphosphate, or ATP. ATP is a usable source of energy for our cells and is the most immediate source of chemical energy for muscular activity.

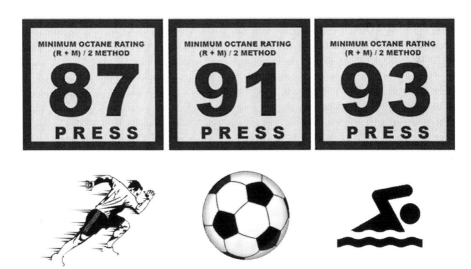

Imagine your body is like a car again. What does a car need to run? Gasoline! There are different grades of gasoline—unleaded, midgrade, and premium. Octane levels are the only difference between the grades of gas, and they are used as a way to impact and improve an engine's performance. The energy systems in our bodies work in a similar way.

We have three energy systems that produce ATP or adenosine triphosphate. The energy systems are called the phosphocreatine system, anaerobic glycolytic system, and the aerobic or oxidative energy system. The first two systems, phosphocreatine and anaerobic glycolytic systems, are both considered anaerobic energy systems, meaning they don't require oxygen to produce ATP. When activities last only a few seconds, your body can produce ATP from the phosphocreatine system. An example of this would be sprinting for 10 seconds or less. When activities last only a few minutes, your body produces ATP from the anaerobic glycolytic system. An example of this would be playing soccer. When activities last longer than a couple of minutes, your body requires oxygen to produce ATP. Your body produces this ATP from your aerobic or oxidative energy system. An example of this would be swimming for an extended period of time.

When oxygen is present, muscles can extract all the available energy from glucose (blood sugar) in about three to 20 minutes of moderate exercise. Your muscles and liver pour out their stored carbohydrates to be used by the muscles. However, the muscles and liver can only store and use a specific amount of glycogen (blood sugar stored in your muscles and liver) before it all runs out.

When you exercise for longer than 20 minutes, you'll need to find another source of fuel to make ATP. After about 20 minutes, the body begins to use less glycogen (blood sugar stored in your muscles and liver) and more and more fat for fuel. Unlike the limited glycogen stores, fat stores can fuel hours of exercise without running out. Body fat is, theoretically, an unlimited source of energy.

Your body wants to use sugar or carbohydrates as the primary source of fuel, but it can also use fat. Unlike a car, our bodies can deplete our glycogen stores (the gasoline) and start burning fat. This usable form of energy in the body is called free fatty acids. Fats taken in through the diet are first digested to produce fatty acids. Then, after these fatty acids are absorbed, they're converted into triglycerides. Triglycerides are stored forms of fatty acids,

When you first start exercising, your blood's fatty acid concentration falls as your muscles begin to draw on these free fatty acids. But if the exercise continues for more than a few minutes, the hormone epinephrine signals the fat cells to break apart so they can be used as energy. After about 20 minutes of exercise, fats or triglycerides are released into the bloodstream to be used as energy. If you work out at the right intensity, fat cells begin to shrink when they empty out their lipid stores. You don't get rid of the fat cell, but you shrink them in size.

Target Heart Rate Zones

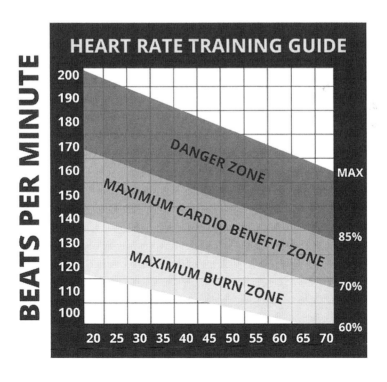

If you go to any gym and read the instructions on the cardio equipment, you'll see references that say if you keep your heart rate at a certain intensity, you'll enter the fat-burning zone. I hate to be the one to tell you, but there is no such thing as a fat-burning zone where you can lose fat efficiently. It's a myth.

Guess what? You actually burn fat the most efficiently when you are sleeping at night. The calories that your body burns while you are sleeping are being pulled directly from your adipose tissue or fat stores. The more active you become, or the higher the intensity of your workout, the less fat you burn. The best way to burn fat effectively is to know which target heart rate zone you should be keeping your heart rate in. This is why many people who just hop on the treadmill end up spinning their wheels and not seeing results. They are just like gerbils on a wheel.

Monitoring your heart rate is one of the most effective methods for measuring and monitoring your exercise intensity, and it's an integral part of our program at PG FIT. You can do this by wearing a heart rate monitor during physical activity. When you have this information, you can tell approximately how intensely you are working out and which heart rate zone you are working in. Your target heart rate is an approximation of where your heart rate should be when you are exercising to improve your cardiorespiratory efficiency and to burn fat. It is going to be different for everyone depending on their age, resting heart rate, and general cardiorespiratory fitness.

There's a basic rule with aerobic exercise. When starting, you should exercise at an intensity that leaves you slightly out of breath but still able to carry on a normal conversation. If you are out of breath and unable to speak, you are becoming oxygen deficient and cannot burn fat.

Often when people do cardio, they work at a really high intensity because they want to burn calories. This poses two problems. First, they are not burning fat calories efficiently. They are burning muscle, which is the last thing you want to burn. Second, they are developing a small aerobic foundation. You can't work on your phosphocreatine system, anaerobic glycolytic system, and aerobic or oxidative energy systems all at once. You have to start by developing an aerobic foundation. To do this, you start by focusing on oxidative energy system first. If you focus too quickly on your anaerobic systems (phosphocreatine and glycolytic systems), you will burn muscle and won't be able to continually improve your aerobic system. This will cause you to plateau, and you will not be able to continually improve all three systems.

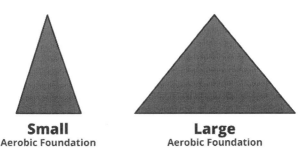

Small
Aerobic Foundation

Large
Aerobic Foundation

Instead, the goal is to start slow and steady and gradually increase the intensity. This will help you develop a large aerobic foundation for improving and maximizing your cardiorespiratory fitness.

Karvonen Formula

Now that you understand the usefulness of heart rate zones, let's determine yours so you can start gaining the benefits. There are five different target heart rate zones. The easiest way to determine your target heart rate zones is to use the Karvonen formula.

The first step is to determine your resting heart rate. Take your right index and middle finger and check your pulse for sixty seconds by applying pressure to your carotid artery in your neck. Your resting heart rate should be somewhere between 60–80 beats per minute. You want to make sure you are calculating your resting heart rate when you are truly at rest. The best time to do this is first thing in the morning.

Once you have calculated your resting heart rate, we want to calculate your maximum heart rate by subtracting your age from

220. So, if you are 50 years old, 220 − 50 = 170. That means your maximum heart rate is 170 beats per minute. This number gives you an approximation of what your maximum heart rate should be. There is a regression formula to figure out what your maximum heart rate should be that is more accurate than the Karvonen formula, but this simple equation is a good place to start. Unfortunately, the only way to know your exact maximum heart is to do some advanced cardio tests. The Karvonen Formula is accurate for about seventy percent of the population, with some room for error, like all tests, so that's why we use the regression formula now.

Once we have calculated your maximum heart rate, we want to determine your heart rate reserve. Your heart rate reserve is the difference between your resting heart rate and your maximum heart rate. This number will help us calculate more accurate target heart rate zones. To get this number, subtract your resting heart rate from your maximum heart rate. For instance, if your resting heart rate is 70 beats per minute, and your maximum heart rate is 170, then 170 − 70 = 100. That means your heart rate reserve is 100 beats per minute.

Now, using your heart rate reserve, we can calculate all five target heart rate zones specifically for you. This is done by multiplying your heart rate reserve by different training zones. The first zone (also called the grey zone) targets a training intensity of 50-60 percent. The second zone (also known as the blue zone) targets a training intensity of 60-70 percent. The third zone (also called the green zone) targets a training intensity of 70-80 percent. The fourth zone (or orange zone) aims for a training intensity of 80-90 percent, and the fifth zone (or red zone) aims for 90-100 percent training intensity.

When you multiply your heart rate reserve by these numbers, you will need to add back in your resting heart rate to make the target heart rate zones more accurate. For instance, if your heart rate reserve is 100 beats per minute, then you'll have 100 x 50% = 50. When you add back the resting heart rate of 70 beats per minute, you'll find 50 + 70 = 120. So, 50 percent of your maximum heart rate is 120 beats per minute.

You would do this with all the other percentages to determine all of the target heart rate zones.

100x60%=60. 60+70=130. 60% is 130 beats per minute.

100x70%=70. 70+70=140. 70% is 140 beats per minute.

100x80%=80. 80+70=150. 80% is 150 beats per minute.

100x90%=90. 90+70=130. 90% is 160 beats per minute.

Once we've done these formulations, we know that the first target heart rate zone of 50–60 percent is 120–130 beats per minute. For someone who is severely deconditioned, this would be the first zone to start in. The second target heart rate zone is 60–70 percent, which is 130–140 beats per minute. This is the heart rate zone where someone who is deconditioned should start. The third target heart rate zone of 70–80 percent is 140–150 beats per minute. Once your heart rate reaches approximately 70–80 percent of your maximum heart rate, this is when you start conditioning your cardiorespiratory system, and you enter your aerobic threshold. Your aerobic threshold is the exertion point where your body is using oxygen to break down sugar (also known as aerobic glycolysis).

The fourth target heart rate zone of 80–90 percent is 150–160 beats per minute. Once your heart rate reaches approximately 80–90 percent of your maximum heart rate, this is when you can start improving your cardiorespiratory system, and you enter your anaerobic threshold. Your anaerobic threshold is the point where oxygen is no longer present, and your body starts pulling energy from your muscles. Once oxygen is no longer present, lactic acid is produced.

The fifth and final target heart rate zone is 90–100 percent, which is 160–170 beats per minute. Getting into your maximum heart rate zone can be very dangerous for a deconditioned client, but once you have developed your aerobic foundation, it can be extremely beneficial to stay in your maximum heart rate zone for short bursts. This is what we call interval training, and it's one of the best ways to maximize your results once you're ready. The goal is to learn how to manipulate all five zones to improve your cardiorespiratory efficiency.

FITTE Principle

Another important concept to understand is what's called the FITTE principle. FITTE is an acronym that stands for frequency, intensity, type, time, and enjoyment. This principle will help you structure a cardiorespiratory program that is appropriate for you.

Frequency is the number of times per week you are going to engage in the cardiorespiratory activity. If someone is deconditioned and they have not been doing cardio for a long time, we recommend that they start doing cardio only a couple of times per week. For an athlete that is looking to improve their cardiorespiratory endurance, they may do cardio five or six times a week.

Intensity is going to be the specific target heart rate zone that you're going to keep your heart rate in while you're doing cardio. There are between two and five target heart rate zones that you want to be able to keep your heart rate in to maximize your results. For a person who is deconditioned or new to cardio, they are going to keep their heart rate in the lower heart rate zones.

You will want to start with light to moderate activity. For someone who is used to doing cardio several days per week, they can work in all five zones.

Type is going to be the mode of cardio you choose to use. There are many different forms of cardio to choose from. It's important to go through a thorough biomechanical assessment to determine if you have any motor dysfunctions, muscle imbalances, or posture deviances that may first need to be addressed. Choosing the wrong mode of cardio can create more of an issue.

Most of our clients have some sort of motor dysfunction, muscle imbalance, or posture deviance. During our biomechanical assessment, we identify these issues and create personalized exercise plans that meet their needs. If, for instance, you have tight hamstrings or lower back issues, you should probably avoid the recumbent bike or rowing machine. Your mode of cardio is going to be dependent on the type of motor dysfunction or muscle imbalances you might have.

For many clients, we recommend beginning with the elliptical trainer. It is low impact, so it's easy on your joints, especially ankles and knees. You can also burn more calories per minute on the elliptical trainer than you can doing many of the other modes of cardio. This is especially true if you're using the arm handles to activate your upper extremity while also working your lower body.

Over time, you can learn proper biomechanics and condition your muscles to work efficiently and effectively. Until that point, you may want to avoid doing multiple forms of cardio or using many different machines. Your body will eventually adapt to the various types of cardio, and you will be able to manipulate this variable later on if you need to.

Time is going to be the duration or how long you're going to do cardio training. As mentioned, you need to be engaged in cardio for a minimum of 20 minutes to start burning fat. When just getting started, most people should participate in cardio activities for a minimum of 20 minutes and a maximum of 60 minutes. If you can do light to moderate intensity for 20 minutes, then you should be able to do cardio for at least 30 to 40 minutes. Your cardio program should total about 40 to 50 minutes. You're going to start with about a five-minute warm-up and gradually increase your heart rate until you get into a target heart rate zone. For 30 to 40 minutes, you will keep your heart rate in this heart rate zone. Then, you will cool down for five minutes and gradually bring your heart rate back down. If you do 40 minutes of cardio plus a five-minute warm-up and a five-minute cooldown, that would be a total duration of 50 minutes.

Enjoyment is the final piece of the puzzle. I don't know too many people, including myself, who enjoy being a hamster on a wheel. I don't like plodding along doing cardio for 40 to 50 minutes. So, I find ways to keep my mind occupied. That's why I'll listen to music, a podcast, a good audiobook, or watch TV so that my mind is occupied while my body is doing the work.

You want to find a way to keep yourself entertained so that you don't think about what you're doing or, worse, try to talk yourself into quitting. The "E" really should stand for entertainment, because you're trying to find a way to keep yourself entertained while making progress. After you finish and the endorphins are released, you'll be glad you did it. While at the end of the day, you may not enjoy doing cardio, it's extremely important if you want to see results.

Physiological Adaptation

It can take up to three to four weeks before you start seeing any improvements. Then, your body will be stronger and have started to adapt physiologically to your new regime. At this point, it's important to restructure your cardio program. You can't keep doing the same activity, because you've gotten stronger and it will no longer stress your cardiorespiratory system or burn fat efficiently. Even taking just a couple of days off and not staying consistent with your cardio program can set you back a couple of weeks. That's why it's extremely important to make sure that you're following a program and staying consistent with it.

There are many assessments and tools you can use to help you determine whether or not you're improving your cardiorespiratory efficiency. We encourage all of our clients to wear a heart rate monitor while they're working out. This way, you can monitor your heart rate and make sure you are working in the right target heart rate zone.

Of all the excellent heart rate monitoring systems, we particularly recommend Polar products. Polar has a straightforward test, called the OwnIndex, that allows you to measure your cardio fitness. First, you download the test via the Polar Beat app. You then put on your heart rate monitor and lay down for three to five minutes while the program analyzes your heart rate.

This is an easy, noninvasive way to measure your cardio fitness. It gives you a number resembling your sub-VO2 Max, which measures the maximum amount of oxygen you can uptake efficiently. The test then gives you a score in milliliters of oxygen per kilogram of body weight per minute or ml/Kg/min. The only way that you can truly measure your VO2 Max is in a clinical setting where you'll wear a breathing apparatus and perform cardio at a very high intensity.

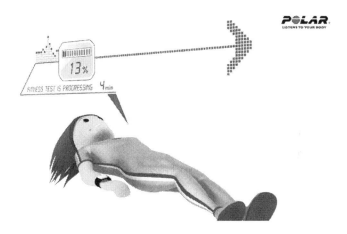

This number is dependent on your age, sex, and cardio fitness. For example, an OwnIndex score below 31 is considered quite low, and a score of 31 to 35 is deemed to be low. Fair is going to be from 36 to 42. Moderate is 43 to 48. Good is from 49 to 53. Very good is 54 to 59, and elite is over 60. These ranges change slightly depending on your age and sex, but they are an excellent guide to follow. You will want to measure your progress every three to four weeks to see whether or not your cardiorespiratory fitness is improving. Measuring your cardio fitness will help you determine how to structure your cardiorespiratory program and how to improve it.

Getting Started

Now, it's time to focus on you. I've included three blank forms in this chapter that you can use to determine your target heart rate zones and your FITTE goals.

If you are new to cardio, you can use the first approach, which simplifies target heart rate zones into two zones. The first zone is light to moderate (about 60 to 80 percent of your maximum heart rate), and the second zone is moderate to hard (about 70 to 90 percent of your maximum heart rate). By focusing on only two zones with a wider range of where you should keep your heart rate, it's a little easier to keep track of things, especially when just getting started.

You still want to keep your heart rate primarily in the light to moderate (60 to 80%) zone. Be sure to write down what the beats per minute should be for both zones.

Age	60-80% of Max HR Light to Moderate	70-90% of Max HR Moderate to Hard
20	120-160	140-180
25	117-156	137-176
30	114-152	133-171
35	111-148	130-167
40	108-144	126-162
45	105-140	123-158
50	102-136	119-153
55	99-132	116-149
60	96-128	112-144
65	93-124	109-140
70	90-120	105-135

Your Personal Target Zones
Target Zone 1
–
Light to Moderate Exercise
Target Zone 2
–
Moderate to Hard Exercise

If you have been following a cardio program for at least three to four weeks, you should use the Cardiorespiratory Program form below to calculate all five target heart rate zones and to structure a cardiorespiratory program. Calculate your resting heart rate, maximum heart rate, and heart rate reserve. Once you have these three numbers, you can calculate the target heart rate zone intensities at 50%, 60%, 70%, 80%, and 90%.

Then, you can use the Polar Beat app to determine your OwnIndex score or VO2 Max, which allows you to create a solid cardio program using the FITTE Principle. Be sure to follow your program for at least three to four weeks and then remeasure your OwnIndex score to see whether or not your cardio fitness is improving.

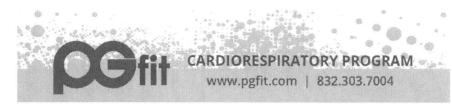

CARDIORESPIRATORY PROGRAM
www.pgfit.com | 832.303.7004

Name:

Age				
Resting Heart Rate				
Maximum Heart Rate				
Heart Rate Reserve				
Target Heart Rate Zones	Intensity			
	50%		bpm	
	60%		bpm	
	70%		bpm	
	80%		bpm	
	AT		bpm	
Activity Level	Beginner			
VO2 MAX				

Notes

Frequency F	2-4x Weekly	
Intensity I	60-70% Zone II	
Type T	Elliptical Trainer	
Time T	5 min warm-up, 20-40 min in correct Zone & a 5 min cool-down	
Enjoyment E	The most important part of following your cardio program is to keep your mind occupied like listening to music or an audio-book, watching TV or your favorite sitcom or talking and working out with a friend or accountability partner.	

How many times a day does your heart beat? This is an important question to ask because the average person has a resting heart rate of about 60 to 80 beats per minute. If you are overweight or obese, your resting heart rate is going to be higher than that. A person's heart usually beats about 115,200 times each day. Just by lowering your heart rate by ten beats per minute, your heart will beat about 14,000 times less per day. That's approximately 5.1 million fewer beats per year and about one-quarter of a billion during your lifetime! That is the equivalent of adding ten years to your life, just by focusing on cardiorespiratory training and lowering your heart rate by ten beats per minute. Do you think it's worth following a structured cardiorespiratory training program now?

CHAPTER 6
Turbocharging Your Results

When I think about the importance of supplements, I always think of a client I trained named Christy. She had been trying to lose weight for several years and was struggling to lose even a few pounds. She had tried a number of different diets and exercise programs but was never successful at losing weight. As a last resort, she decided to start working with a personal trainer and contacted me.

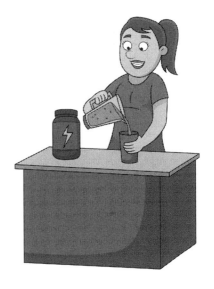

For the first few weeks that she worked with me, she struggled to lose any weight. At first, I thought that it had to do with her diet. But I knew she was being honest about logging her food and tracking how many calories she was taking in. She was also putting in the hard work at the gym. She followed a structured cardio program a few days a week and did a form of resistance training with me three times a week. After about a month of doing this, she was not losing any weight. She became very discouraged and wanted to quit. But there was one thing we had not reviewed.

We decided to look at her micronutrient profile to see whether or not she was getting all the vitamins and minerals she needed from her diet. We found that she was not getting the Recommended Dietary Allowance (RDA) for several micronutrients. In fact, Christy was severely deficient in calcium because she was avoiding dairy. She had heard it was bad for you, but she was not eating enough other calcium-rich foods (like spinach, kale, beans, fish, etc.) to make up the difference.

Among other things, calcium helps with fat oxidation. It helps break up fat so that it can be utilized as energy. Because Christy was calcium deficient, she was not able to metabolize fat or lose weight. Once she started taking a calcium supplement—along with a multivitamin and protein powder—she lost a few pounds within the first week. Do you think Christy became motivated at this point? You bet!

She had been creating such a caloric and micronutrient deficit that her body was robbing her bones and muscles of available nutrients instead of burning fat. After several months of taking the right supplements, she was able to get to her goal weight. This is one of many examples of clients who have added supplements to help turbocharge their results.

When I first started in the industry, I did not believe in the importance of supplements. I thought they were a rip-off. I had spent thousands of dollars on supplements and didn't see any difference in my physique. I was eating and working out the same as always, and I thought the supplements would give me the boost I needed. They didn't. It wasn't until I was trying to build lean muscle mass that I discovered not all supplements are equal. Once I was able to get on a quality protein and amino acid supplement, I started to see striation in my muscles that I had never seen before.

You might ask yourself why you should need to take supplements. When you're trying to lose weight, you are creating what's called a caloric deficit. To create a caloric deficit, you have to eat less by cutting some food out of your diet. When you create a caloric deficit, you're also creating what's called a micronutrient deficit. It's important to make sure you're getting all the vitamins and minerals your body needs—but without the calories.

The problem with the supplement industry is that the FDA does not regulate it. In 1994, the Dietary Supplement Health and Education Act (DSHEA) was signed. It states that the FDA is not authorized to review dietary supplement products for safety and effectiveness before they are marketed. Dietary supplements are not subject to the safety and efficacy testing requirements that drugs are. What does that mean? The supplement industry is like the Wild West. There might be a sheriff in town, but anything goes unless a law is broken. In this case, someone usually has to die before that happens.

What Is a Supplement?

A supplement, by definition, can be anything that enhances your diet or food intake. Supplements are anything that is taken to add extra nutrients or to replace missing nutrients. Supplements can be vitamins, minerals, amino acids, fatty acids, herbs, or many other substances and can be delivered in the form of a pill, tablet, capsule, liquid, and so forth. Supplements are essential because they help replace the micronutrients that you are not getting from the food you're eating.

There are two types of micronutrients. Vitamins are the first type and are vital organic dietary supplements. Vitamins cannot be made or produced inside the body. They are important for regulating a variety of everyday biological functions. They are not actual food and don't supply energy. Within the vitamin category, there are two types—water- and fat-soluble vitamins. Vitamins A, D, E, and K are fat-soluble, while vitamins B and C are water-soluble.

The other group of micronutrients is minerals. Minerals are essential control agents for making hormones and enzymes, and are necessary for energy production, cell reproduction, and body maintenance. Like vitamins, minerals also do not supply your body with energy. There are two types of minerals—major and trace minerals. Calcium, phosphorus, sodium, and potassium are examples of major minerals. Magnesium, iron, and zinc are a few examples of trace minerals.

The USDA has stated that less than one percent of the American population gets all of the micronutrients they need daily. Even if you could eat all the right kinds of foods, it's still virtually impossible to get all the micronutrients our bodies need. One reason for this is that the soil isn't as nutrient dense as it once was. In 1951, a woman could get the Recommended Dietary Allowance (RDA) of vitamin A from one peach. Today, a woman would have to eat several peaches just to get the same RDA for vitamin A. We have also introduced over 70,000 chemicals into our environment in the form of herbicides, pesticides, fungicides, and larvicides, just to name a few. These chemicals affect the nutritional value of our food when it's processed.

Many illnesses and diseases are a result of a deficiency in one or more vitamins and minerals. We could cure many of these ailments if we would eat right and take the right supplements to enhance our diets.

What to Look For

The world of nutritional supplements is confusing. There are so many items to choose from, and all of them claim to be the very best. Not all supplements are created equal, though. Be careful not to fall for gimmicks or false advertising. If it sounds too good to be true, it probably is.

If you've ever seen a supplement advertisement, you probably noticed that skin or sex appeal is frequently used in the ad to sell the product. Sometimes it doesn't matter how good a product is—the right advertising tactics can sell it. Conversely, you could have the best product, but if you can't market it, it will never be able to compete in the supplement world!

Supplements are often abused and misused. And there are many supplements on the market that have the potential to do more harm to your body than good. Many contain fillers, contaminants, and even carcinogens—all of which can be detrimental to your health.

When you're trying to decide which supplements to buy, there are a few important things to look for. For example, does a licensed pharmaceutical manufacturer make the product? If so, it will likely have gone through some pretty stringent testing to ensure safety and efficacy. With any supplement, you want the product to have a United States Pharmacopoeia Verified (USP) or Good Manufacturing Practices (GMP) mark or label.

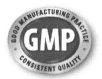

The USP Verified mark on a supplement label indicates that the product contains the ingredients in the declared potency and amounts as listed on the label. It also indicates that the product does not contain harmful levels of specified contaminants, which almost all supplements have at least traces of. It also confirms that the supplement will break down and release into the body within a specified amount of time. Most supplements should breakdown in the small intestines because that is where most micronutrients are digested.

A GMP registration assures a supplement has the identity, strength, composition, quality, and purity that appear on its label. GMP testing is usually done on a sample batch of products rather than all, so it's not as stringent a process as a those that receive a USP Verified mark. But it still gives the user better information than no product testing at all. I always recommend investing in the highest quality product your budget will allow. With lesser-quality products, you can never know what exactly might be in them.

For any supplement you choose, you should also look for any published scientific (not anecdotal) studies on humans. This information is not always available since most of the studies done about supplements are conducted on mice. Data on the effects of these products on mice is only marginally useful since mice have only 1/10,000th of their DNA in common with human beings.

You also need to be careful when using multiple supplements or using products from multiple manufacturers. An individual product may have trace levels of potentially harmful ingredients but still be considered in the safe range. But when combined with other products (or the same product from another manufacturer) you may reach unsafe levels.

If you are taking medications or prescriptions, you should always consult with a pharmacist before you take any supplements. A pharmacist will have a Physicians Desk Reference (PDR) that they can use to check to see if there are any possible synergistic or antagonistic effects that could result from combining supplements with your prescriptions or any over-the-counter medications you may be taking.

Getting Started

When starting a supplement plan, here's what I think is important. First, take a good quality multivitamin. It should be taken with food at intervals throughout the day. Two of the most popular multivitamins on the market are Centrum and One-A-Day.

Many studies show that your body only absorbs a small fraction of the micronutrients in these brands of pills, and most of the nutrients are eliminated from your system. You want to make sure to take a multivitamin that will be absorbed into your body, not eliminated through your urine or feces. That's why it's important to look for a brand or manufacturer that has a GMP or USP Verified mark.

The next supplement that I recommend is a quality protein supplement or meal replacement shake. These will likely contain hydrolyzed whey protein and be loaded with Branched Chain Amino Acids (BCAAs) and other amino acids to help build and repair your muscles. The reason that you want to use a hydrolyzed whey protein shake, powder, or liquid is that hydrolyzed means it has been partially broken down. It contains predigested enzymes to break down the protein into amino acids faster so that it can be quickly absorbed into your bloodstream and used as energy.

When you eat a complete protein, like a chicken breast, for example, it will take your body at least three hours to metabolize it as a usable source of energy. Immediately following your workout, you want to make sure to replenish your body with carbohydrates and amino acids. These protein supplements and shakes are also a quick and convenient way to supplement one of your meals, especially if you're on the go all the time.

In addition to those found in protein powders, shakes, etc., I also would recommend a supplement of BCAAs before or after a workout. Your muscle fibers are nutrient-dense, and they contain water, vitamins, minerals, electrolytes, and protein. About 50 to 60 percent of the content in your muscles is made up of three amino acids—leucine, isoleucine, and valine. BCAAs are considered essential because unlike some (nonessential) amino acids, your body cannot make them. Therefore, it is necessary to get them from your diet.

BCAAs play several other roles in your body too. They not only help build protein and muscle, but also regulate blood sugar levels and help reduce the fatigue you feel during exercise by reducing the production of serotonin in your brain.

Calcium is the next supplement I recommend. Why? Well, it's one of the most essential minerals in your diet, and it's necessary for life. According to the surgeon general, more than 10 million Americans over the age of 50 have osteoporosis, and 34 million are at risk. Calcium not only helps build strong bones, but it also enables our blood to clot, our muscles to contract, and our heart to beat. Calcium is also critical for weight management, helping with fat oxidation. Remember what it did for Christy?

The RDA for calcium is 1,000 milligrams daily for adults. I believe you should strive to get at least 1,500 milligrams each day, but you need to be careful not to take too much. It's important to make sure you take the right kind of calcium and other micronutrients like vitamin D, magnesium, and zinc to aid in the digestion of the calcium.

An omega complex is also a good supplement to incorporate into your daily routine. Omega-3 fatty acids are vital for healthy development and growth. Since the human body cannot make omega-3 fatty acids, we have to get them from our diet. They can help prevent and treat many serious diseases. There is evidence that they can aid in heart health, and they also help support healthy brain function.

Omega-6 fatty acids are healthy in the right amounts, but too much is believed to be a significant contributing factor for many diseases, especially cardiovascular disease. Omega-9 fatty acids are not essential. They are produced by the body and are the most abundant fats in most cells in the body with many beneficial health effects.

There is no official Recommended Dietary Allowance for omega-3 fatty acids, but most health organizations agree that 250–500 milligrams per day of combined EPA and DHA is enough for adults to maintain overall health. I recommend taking at least 1,000 milligrams of an omega complex that contains omega-3, -6, and -9 in the right ratios. Since we generally eat enough omega -6 and -9 in our diets, I would recommend taking an omega complex that will have twice as much omega-3 as compared to -6 and -9.

These are just a few of the supplements that we recommend starting with because they are generally the micronutrients that many of our clients are lacking in their diet. There are other supplements that we would recommend, like a probiotic or antioxidant. If you want to take other supplements, specifically goals enhancers like fat burners or muscle building products, you should try the most natural approach before using any genetically altered compounds.

Some of the most common supplements are fat burners or thermogenics. These products raise your core temperature. Some of the most common muscle-building supplements are creatine or testosterone boosters. Please be careful if you decide to use products like these because they have been genetically altered. They can change your body's chemistry, hormones, and bodily functions. If you take them for too long, they can also cause long-term damage and impede you from seeing results.

There are many consumer reports that show how harmful some of the leading supplements are. Some of them contain arsenic, cadmium, lead, mercury, and other toxins and impurities. You want to make sure that you're very careful about what supplements you are taking. Remember, the supplement industry can be like the Wild West, so you have to be very cautious and look for products that contain a USP Verified mark or GMP label. Additionally, I recommend that you try to find natural supplements rather than taking something that's been genetically altered.

Supplement Questionnaire

Below is a supplement questionnaire that can help you determine which micronutrients you might be deficient in and the supplements you might want to consider.

As I have mentioned, I can't emphasize enough the importance of eating whole foods and consuming plenty of vegetables and fruit. Food needs to be our first source of fuel. However, it's virtually impossible to get all the micronutrients we need from whole food anymore. We should supplement in addition to or in replacement of whole foods that we are not getting through our diet.

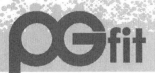

SUPPLEMENT
WORKSHEET

Name:		
Yes	No	
		Do you take a multivitamin daily?
		Are you currently consuming three to four servings of calcium or at least 1000mg of calcium each day?
		Do you regularly eat 12-14 servings of fruits and vegetables each day or take an antioxidant?
		Do you take a probiotic?
		Are you currently consuming 25-35 grams of fiber each day?
		Are you currently consuming three to five servings of fish or seafood each week or take a 1000mg of fish, krill or flaxseed oil daily?
		Do you drink caffeine or take other stimulants each day? QTY
		Do you currently take supplements like BCAA, Amino Acids, protein bars or shakes?
		Do you currently take other supplements or goal enhancers?
		Do you know what GMP or USP stands for on a supplement label?

Supplement Recommendations

1. A good multivitamin is designed to be taken at intervals throughout the day. You should take a multi-vitamin at least two times a day with food.

2. If you don't consume three to four serving of dairy each day, you should consider taking at least 1000 mg of calcium like the PG Fit MagCalZinc.

3. If you don't eat enough fruits and vegetables, you should consider taking an antioxidant like Reserve.

4. A probiotic will help restore your body with healthy bacteria. You should consider taking a probiotic each day, like acidophilus.

5. If you are not consuming 25-35 grams of fiber each day, you should consider taking a fiber supplement, like psyllium husk.

6. If you don't consume at least 3-5 servings of seafood each week, you should consider taking a 1000-3000 mg of an omega complex each day, like the PG Fit Salmon Oil.

7. If you drink more than 1 serving of a caffeinated beverage each day, you should consider cutting you caffeine intake to less than 80 mg each day.Caffeine can have synergist or antagonist affects on supplements meaning it can slow down or speed up the rate of absorption of nutrients in your body.

8. You should consider drinking at least one high quality protein shake each day, like the Zen Fuze. You should also consider using a high-quality protein bar, like Power Crunch, Think Thin or Oatmega to fill in the gap in between meals. If you workout consistently, you should also consider taking BCAAs, like Zen Fit, after your workout.

9. You want to be careful if you take any other supplements, besides the ones we have listed. You can reach the upper levels of toxicity by taking more supplements than your body needs. Please consult with a qualified physician before you start a dietary support or supplement program.

10. Not all supplements are created equally. Supplements are not regulated by the FDA, so be sure to use high-quality supplements. that follow Good Manufacturing Practices (GMP) or have the US Pharmacopiea verified mark. We recommend the PG Fit supplements as well as those manufactured by Jeunesse, Bluebonnet, Nature's Plus and NOW.

If you answer "No" to any of the questions above, see the recommendations below the questions. If you are not used to taking supplements, it might be a little overwhelming to go through and answer the questions. Remember, balance and moderation are key.

If you are not taking any supplements currently, start with a good-quality multivitamin. Once you consistently take a multivitamin, then you can add in a quality protein supplement or meal replacement shake. Start with these two supplements and be sure to eat plenty of vegetables and fruits.

CHAPTER 7

How to Turn Your Body into a Fat-Burning Machine

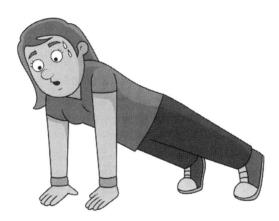

My first experience with weight training was in the high school weight room when I played football. My football coaches were not very well educated on the importance of weight training, and their idea of weight training was to have the team bench, squat, and deadlift as much as we could. This was a recipe for disaster. One day, I was doing a chest press with dumbbells heavier than I weighed at the time. My arms started giving out. As I went to set them down, my finger got wedged between the dumbbell and a metal plate leaning up against the bench, and I cut the tip of my finger off. Blood started squirting from the top of my finger, and I was rushed to the emergency room to get my fingertip sewn back on.

After that, I was hesitant to do any heavy weightlifting because I didn't feel like I knew what I was doing. I would occasionally do some weight training, but it was mostly what was called dryland training. We would do a lot of push-ups, pull-ups, squats, lunges, and of course, core work. I would lift weights occasionally at a gym, but I never really lifted heavy again.

Resistance Training

I didn't really understand the importance of resistance training until I started working with a strength and conditioning coach when I was in college. That was the first time I was introduced to a new world of weight training—one I never knew existed. It was the first time I was given a structured weight training program that was based on a series of assessments and tests. I was shown how to do the exercises correctly and coached through the workout. I had a program designed specifically to show me what exercises I was supposed to do, in what order, and how many sets and repetitions of each exercise I was supposed to do. I even knew how long I was supposed to rest before I started the next lift.

When I became a certified personal trainer and started training at a gym, I would watch people come into the facility who were just as confused as I had been when I first started weight training in high school. Most people don't have a clue about what they should be doing when they begin weight training.

I observed that most people would only use the machines they were familiar with and would go through a circuit using just that equipment. Then they would repeat that same circuit each time they came in. They would typically do three sets of 10–15 repetitions and rest for two to three minutes in between sets. This is one of the most ineffective ways to weight train.

I would also observe individuals who would lift heavy—like I use to do in high school—and would be so sore that they often wouldn't come back in for a few weeks. Or worse, they would injure themselves and be out of commission even longer. You shouldn't be so sore that you can't move. It's estimated that 80 percent of the population has lower back pain or other joint or connective tissue problems. The worst thing you can do when you have pain is lifting heavy weights. Pain is not always an indicator of a good workout. There is a big difference between a little bit of muscle soreness and joint or acute pain.

Resistance training can be anything from bodyweight exercises to machine-based exercises. There are so many different forms of resistance training, and it can be hard to determine which form of training is right for you.

The simple answer is that all resistance training has value. Resistance or weight training is particularly important for burning body fat. Fat is burned inside your muscles. When you activate your muscles and, more importantly, increase your lean muscle mass, you turn your body into a fat-burning machine. This is how you start sculpting your body—you build muscle mass and begin to get rid of fat that is covering your muscle. Together, these result in more definition, helping you achieve the body you've always dreamed of.

Are You Training or Exercising?

I always like to ask this question: Which one weighs more muscle or fat? If you had one pound of muscle and one pound of fat, which one would weigh more? The answer should be obvious. They would weigh the same. However, most people think that muscle weighs more than fat. One pound is one pound. The difference is that muscle is denser. It has a smaller volume. If you had the same volume of fat and the same volume of muscle, the muscle would weigh more.

But like I said, one pound is one pound. Most people have a hard time building muscle and losing body fat at the same time. The average person can only gain about a quarter of a pound to one pound of lean muscle mass in any given month. The goal is to turn your body into a fat-burning machine. By increasing the amount of lean muscle you have, you're going to be able to start burning fat efficiently.

When most people go to the gym, they go to exercise. They are only concerned about what kind of effect they can have on their body that day. Anyone can exercise. Exercise is just a physical activity. It's a workout to produce a result for that day—burning calories, increasing heart rate, etc. There is nothing wrong with exercising. It beats sitting on the couch.

But what you need to start thinking about is training. Training is a physical activity done with a longer-term goal in mind. Training involves a series of workouts which are specifically designed to attain a certain goal. If you want to turn your body into a fat-burning machine, you can't just go to the gym and exercise. You have to start training with a purpose, and that purpose needs to be to strengthen and tone your muscles.

So how does resistance training turn your body into a fat-burning machine? Some basic math calculations can answer that. One pound of fat burns approximately two to four calories throughout the day. One pound of muscle, on the other hand, can burn up to 90 calories a day, with the average being approximately 50 calories per day. Of course, this all depends on a number of facts, like where the muscle tissue is located and how active it is.

But to keep the math simple, if you were to gain 10 pounds of muscle, you could burn an extra 500 calories a day (10 x 50 = 500). And if you were to sustain that over seven days, that equates to 3,500 calories, which is one pound of fat loss.

Now I know that 10 pounds of muscle may seem like a lot, but it's actually possible over time if you follow the right training program. An important thing to remember is that you can't spot reduce, but you can spot gain. You can increase the size and strength of your muscles in desired locations, but you can't tell your body where to lose fat. If you want to see leaner hips, butt, and thighs, just doing exercises that isolate those areas of your body will not cause you to lose fat in those areas. In fact, you might even gain inches in those areas.

Women often think that if they strength train, they will get big and bulky. But that's not true. Women are built for hyperplasia, not hypertrophy. Hyperplasia means that women can increase the strength and size of their connective tissues, like their tendons and ligaments, not their muscles. Hypertrophy means that you can increase the size of your muscles, which is easy for men. Hormonally, women are not built to get big and bulky. It can be challenging for women to increase the size of their muscle fibers. That's why strength training is so necessary. Women have to strength train in order to strengthen and tone their muscles; otherwise, they will lose what muscle tissue they have.

Anaerobic Training

Resistance training is also called anaerobic training. Anaerobic means that it does not require oxygen to be present in order to produce energy. The energy source, adenosine triphosphate or ATP, is the most immediate source of chemical energy for muscular activity. If you suddenly jumped two feet into the air from a standing start or sprinted 40 yards, the energy source you would be using is ATP from your phosphocreatine system. ATP is stored in most cells, particularly muscle cells. With resistance training, two systems are responsible for making ATP—phosphocreatine and the anaerobic glycolytic systems.

An activity that occurs in less than 10 seconds relies on the phosphocreatine system. ATP is produced through a chemical compound known as phosphocreatine that is stored in the muscles. Any type of ballistic, sprint, or high-intensity exercise, like jumping or sprinting, lasting less than 10 seconds uses this system. The body must find another source after the first 10 seconds. For activities longer than 10 seconds and up to a few minutes, muscles rely on the next available fuel source—the anaerobic glycolytic system—to replenish ATP during exercise. An example of this would be playing soccer, because you are jogging, sprinting, and stopping.

Technically, the anaerobic glycolytic system is also known as the lactic acid system. Anaerobic glycolysis is the breakdown of sugar or carbohydrates without oxygen. In this system, the breakdown of sugar supplies the necessary energy required to resynthesize ATP. However, when carbohydrates are only partially broken down, lactic acid is produced—the reason it's also called the lactic acid system. Lactic acid is what causes the burning sensation in your muscles when you're working out. It's important to follow a resistance training program that will manipulate both of these energy systems to help you see the best results possible.

Another thing that's important to understand is that you have different types of muscle fibers. You have quick twitch, intermediate twitch, and slow endurance twitch muscle fibers. It's important to make sure that you're activating these different types of muscle fibers throughout the workout. An experienced trainer can develop a program that will help maximize your workout.

Resistance training is a very complex and technical process. To help you understand it, I want you to think of a chocolate chip cookie. I love chocolate chip cookies! When I was growing up, my father made the best chocolate chip cookies. It wasn't until many years later 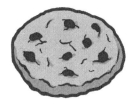 that I realized one of the reasons his cookies were better than any other chocolate chip cookies I'd had is because they were made with "butter-flavored" Crisco.

What are the ingredients for a chocolate chip cookie? There are many, like flour, chocolate chips, sugar, vanilla extract, eggs, and baking soda. And you need an oil or butter—or, in my dad's case, Crisco—to bind it all together. Following the recipe is important. If you use more flour than the recipe calls for, your cookies are going to be hard and flat. I know this because I've learned the hard way. If you use more sugar than indicated in the recipe, the cookies are going to taste sweeter than usual. Everybody likes chocolate, but if you use more chocolate chips than the recipe calls for, they taste better, right? They might. But the cookies also might not hold together. If you do not use the correct measurement for each ingredient and add each element in the correct order, it's going to alter the recipe and the way the cookies will look and taste.

Well, it's the same thing when you're developing a resistance training program to increase muscle mass. Just like there are certain ingredients in a cookie recipe, there are certain variables that you need to consider when you're designing a resistance training program. The first one is workout selection. The program that you select needs to be specific to what you're trying to accomplish. The second consideration is the number of sets you do. The third is the number of repetitions you're going to perform of each set.

The fourth thing to consider is the tempo or the time that it takes to do a repetition. This can be one of the most critical parts of the exercise because the length of time under tension can significantly affect the outcome you're trying to accomplish. The fifth consideration is the intensity or the amount of weight that you're using. It's crucial that you are lifting the right amount of weight to overload your muscles beyond what they are already used to doing. The last variable is the rest period, or how long you should rest in between exercises or sets.

If you add in the benefits of cardiorespiratory (aerobic) training in between resistance training sets, you can maximize your results, especially if you make sure you keep your heart rate in the right target heart rate zone. It's important to look at all the variables because these factors determine what phase of training you're working in and what the outcome will be. Just like the ingredients in a cookie recipe, these training variables will determine what kind of results you will see. Working with a trainer is the best way to make sure you have a program that balances all of these elements.

One of the things that I appreciate about the fitness industry is that it's continually evolving. The more we learn about the human body, the more our training methods should be based on science and research. I often wonder why there are still so many different training modalities and styles out there that are not backed by scientific data to support their methods.

If you start doing something that you haven't done before, you will stress the body and the body will adapt and hopefully become bigger and stronger. But does this mean that it is an effective training program or right for you? Of course not! Don't you want to learn how to work out the right way and as efficiently as possible?

Integrated Training

At PG Fit, we follow a very scientific and cohesive approach. There are two systems that we use together—we call it Functional Integrated Training. The first system is called the Optimum Performance Training Model, or OPT Model, which was developed by the National Academy of Sports Medicine. The other model we follow is called the Functional Movement System, or FMS.

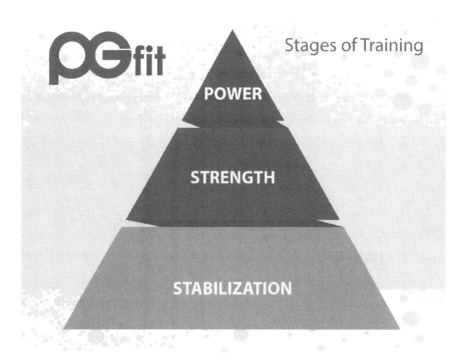

Within the OPT model, there are different stages and phases of training. The first stage is called stabilization; the second is strength; and the third stage is power. Each stage has a purpose. They build on each other, and it can take several weeks to several months to progress from one stage to the next. Within the stages of training, there are also phases of training. The first phase is what we call Corrective Exercise Training. The second phase is Stabilization Endurance Training. The third phase is called Strength Endurance Training. The fourth phase is Hypertrophy. The fifth phase is Maximum Strength Training, and the sixth phase is called Power Training.

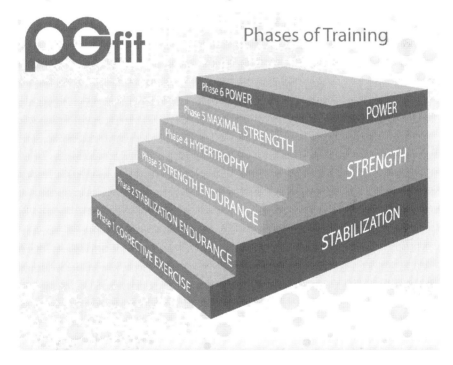

There is an additional phase of training (not included in the chart) that is specific to an athlete or someone who wants to improve or enhance their performance for a particular sport. It's called Sports Specific or Performance Enhancement Training. There has been a lot of research and scientific data to support the validity of this training mode, which is why we use it when working with athletes versus trying to develop one on our own.

The other model we follow is called the Functional Movement System or FMS. The Functional Movement System is a model that was designed to focus on the importance of movement. Most of the time, when personal trainers design training programs, they focus on isolating specific muscle groups. I used to do this as well until I meet Gray Cook, cofounder of FMS.

Working with him, I learned that all of our muscles either work together synergistically or oppose one another antagonistically. It's important to design training programs that focus on specific movement patterns instead of just isolating particular muscles, so muscles work together in an integrated fashion. There are seven different movement patterns that we perform every day, and that's why the training program is called the Functional Movement System.

At PG Fit, we have developed a program called Functional Integrated Training that uses both the OPT Model and FMS. It is a system that follows the scientific and integrated approach developed by these two models. This system will help you maximize your results. The program we develop for you will focus on helping you progress through specific stages and phases of training, and will incorporate movements or exercises that are functional to things that you do every day.

When most people go to the gym, they follow a traditional strength training program, using machines or different pieces of sectorized equipment. Most of this equipment is designed to isolate specific muscle groups instead of focusing on everyday movements. The problem is that this is typically one of the most ineffective ways to train because you're only working one or two muscle groups—not integrating as many muscle groups as possible. How often do you lay down and press something like you would during a bench press? Not very often!

I'm not saying that a bench press never has a place in training. When you're following a hypertrophy program and are trying to increase the size and strength of your muscle fibers, doing bench presses is a good way to isolate your pectoralis major muscles. But for overall results, this should only be one phase of training and not the main emphasis of your weight training program. If you go to the gym on National Chest Day (or any Monday), everyone is working their chest. Is this the right way to work out? We don't think so.

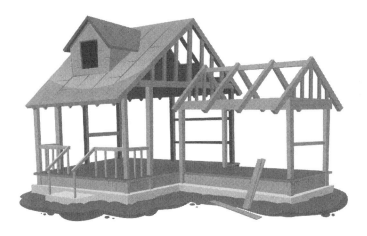

The Optimum Performance Training model is a lot like building a house. Imagine you were building a new home to live in. The first thing you would need to do is to pour the foundation and complete all the electrical and plumbing work. This is the purpose of Stabilization Endurance training or the first phase of stabilization training. You need to start stabilizing the core and activating and strengthening all the connective tissues that surround your joints.

Then you would need to start framing and drywalling the house. This is what the second phase of training is like—Strength Endurance training. You need to start activating and integrating your muscle groups. This is one of my personal favorite forms of training because you get the benefits of stabilization training while you begin to focus on strength training. Did I mention that it's also very efficient?

When most people start a resistance training program, they jump right into the strength or power stages of training. They'll begin to follow some form of a Hypertrophy or Maximal Strength Training program, where they're doing anywhere from three to five sets of six to twelve repetitions, and resting for one to five minutes in between sets. This is precisely what I did all those years ago in high school athletics, and there are several problems with starting a program like this. You are trying to roof the house and paint it without going through all the proper steps of building the house—like pouring the foundation, completing the plumbing and electrical work, or framing and drywalling. As a result, people often injure themselves within the first few weeks of this sort of program (like I did).

Before you develop a resistance training program, you should undergo a biomechanical assessment. This is something we do for every new PG Fit client. It helps to determine if there are any motor dysfunctions, muscle imbalances, or posture deviances that might affect the ability to do certain movements or lifts. We all develop motor dysfunctions and muscle imbalances. This can happen when muscles are not activating the way they should, and other muscle groups have to help out to do the movement or exercise.

For example, many people do push-ups incorrectly. Instead of activating the pectoralis major, which is the main muscle group that should be working, they're activating their shoulders or trapezius or other muscles that shouldn't be activated during a push-up. They are also not working or engaging muscle groups like their core or glutes. As a result, they often feel the exercise in their shoulders or lower back because they are compensating.

What is the Most Important Part of a Workout?

Flexibility training is arguably the most important part of a workout. Several years ago, I met a client who couldn't walk without pain. She had met with several specialists, including an orthopedic surgeon, chiropractor, and massage therapist, to help her with her debilitating pain. No one was able to ease her discomfort.

Every time she walked, her right leg hurt, and as a last resort, she sought the help of a personal trainer. I had an opportunity to provide her biomechanical assessment, and I noticed a few dysfunctions in her movements. I began by designing a flexibility routine for her to follow. We spent the entire session stretching. By the end of our session, she walked out without pain for the first time in a long time. I didn't do anything magical to help her. But her muscles had been so tight that they were impinging on her nerves, stressing her tendons and ligaments, and causing joint dysfunction.

Flexibility training involves three very distinct parts. The first is soft tissue work or Self Myofascial Release (SMFR). SMFR is something you should do before you start working out and at the very end of your workout. It's common to develop tightness or knots in muscles and fascia. SMFR is a process to help you break up the adhesions resulting from microscopic tears in your muscles. It's often performed on a foam roller.

Our muscle spindles are similar to a rubber band. They have a lot of elasticity and flexibility. If you tie a rubber band into a knot, it loses a lot of its spring. You'll find that if you shoot it, it won't go very far. But, if you take the knot out, the rubber band will go farther and faster. Similarly, what happens if you put a rubber band in the freezer and then try to fling it? It will likely break. Our muscles work the same way. The last thing you want to do is stretch your muscles without properly warming up and working out the knots.

The second part of flexibility training involves lengthening and activating your muscles. This can be done through a form of stretching known as active isolated stretching or more familiarly known as corrective exercises. Corrective exercises are important to help overcome motor dysfunctions or muscle imbalances. They are also important to help you warm up, preparing your body for the workout that day.

The third part of flexibility training is making sure you go through a static stretching program at the end of the workout to elongate your muscles, helping to get them back to their proper length-tension relationship. Static means that you hold the stretch in a still or isolated position for at least 20 to 30 seconds.

All three types of flexibility training exercises are important when working out. But they are often overlooked or omitted because of time constraints. As you get older, your workout may even consist mostly of these three parts, because having a proper range of motion and movement in exercises is key to an effective workout. Failure to train for flexibility can lead to motor dysfunctions or muscle imbalances, which makes it difficult to exercise correctly.

The Functional Movement System

The FMS focuses on seven key movement patterns. These are the same movement patterns that we evaluate during the biomechanical assessment to determine whether movements are performed without limitations or compensations. We have simplified the system by using colors to identify each movement pattern. The seven screenings are designed to determine if you have any motor dysfunctions or muscle imbalances that can be identified while the movement is performed. It helps us identify probable overactive and underactive muscle groups that can cause dysfunction or altered movement during the screening. Following are the movements and their corresponding colors.

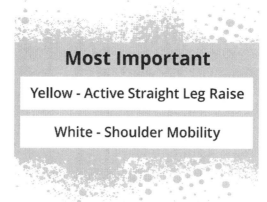

Most Important

Yellow - Active Straight Leg Raise

White - Shoulder Mobility

Second Most Important

Orange - Rotary Stability

Red - Torso Stability Push-Up

Functional Movements

Blue - In-Line Lunge

Green - Hurdle Step

Purple - Overhead Deep Squat

There is a hierarchy regarding the movement patterns, so our assessments are done in a specific order. We start by looking at asymmetrical movements and then assess symmetrical movements. In simple terms, we want to look at each side of the body independently before starting to look at compound or multi-joint movements. We assign a color to any movement that needs to be addressed before proceeding with exercises targeting that area.

The first movement we look at is the active straight leg raise (yellow color). If someone has any sort of hip dominant issue or tightness, we'll have the client refrain from doing deadlifts or other hip dominant exercises.

The second movement pattern assessed is shoulder mobility (white color). If a client has any shoulder mobility limitations, we have them refrain from doing certain shoulder exercises and from pressing overhead.

The third movement pattern we look at is rotary stability (orange color). If a person has any asymmetries in their core or has difficulty stabilizing their core, we won't have them do any advanced core exercises or running until the issue is remedied.

The next movement pattern addressed is the torso stability push-up (red color). If a person has a problem engaging their core or glute musculature and has trouble doing a push-up, we refrain from having them do push-ups or planks on the floor.

The last three movement patterns are more compound or complex movements. The first one is the in-line lunge (blue color). If a person has difficulty performing this movement, we have them avoid doing exercises that include lunge moves.

The sixth movement pattern is the hurdle step (green color). If a person has difficulty performing a hurdle step, we will prevent them from running and jumping, as well as from doing advanced single-leg exercises.

The final movement pattern we assess is the overhead deep squat (purple color). If a person has a difficult time performing an overhead deep squat, we have them refrain from doing any resisted squatting or jumping.

The chart below provides a quick and easy reference, by color, for activities to avoid when you have been assessed to have issues or limitations in a movement area (or areas).

Red Light List

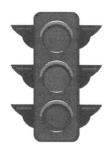

Exercises to Avoid Temporarily

If you have been given a color for one of the seven movement patterns, please review which exercises from the red light lists you should avoid.

Yellow – Active Straight Leg Raise

No deadlifting or hip dominant exercises

White – Shoulder Mobility

No overhead shoulder exercises

Orange – Rotary Stability

No advanced core exercises or running

Red – Torso Stability Push Up

No push-ups or planks on floor

Blue – In-Line Lunge

No lunges

Green – Hurdle Step

No running, jumping, or advanced single leg exercises

Purple – Overhead Deep Squat

No resisted squatting or jumping

It's important to address the movement patterns in the correct order—the order they appear in above. Yellow and White are the most important corrections to address first, followed by the remaining colors. Just by cleaning up your weakest links, you should be able to improve other movement patterns.

A motor dysfunction occurs when the nervous system does not allow a muscle to activate or fire the way it should. A muscle imbalance often results from one muscle group being short and more than likely tight while another muscle group is stretched out and more than likely weak. Motor dysfunctions and muscle imbalances can lead to postural distortion patterns, which can create a number of problems when motions are repeated in a workout.

For example, just one motor dysfunction in the foot/ankle complex can affect the way your muscles activate and the way your joints move. In turn, these can alter your movement and posture. We see clients with neck pain, but the problem originated in their feet. The human body is a very interconnected system—one slight imbalance can cause compensatory effects throughout your entire body.

When it comes to working out, the most important thing you can do is to learn to "crawl before you run"—start slowly with the right developmental patterns and build on a solid foundation. That's why when we design programs, whether it's for our personal training clients or a group, we want to make sure that they're following a structured program that's appropriate for them. We incorporate periodization schemes into the plans we develop, sequencing the exercises so that each time you work out, you're slowly making progress.

Foam Rolling for Healthy Muscles

On the next few pages, I have provided you with some foam rolling techniques, corrective exercises, and stretches. These can and should be done frequently to help keep muscles healthy and flexible.

Using a foam roller is one of the best self-myofascial release exercises you can do to improve the quality of your muscle tissue. The foam roller will increase blood flow to the muscles and help to work out "knots." It gives you many of the benefits of static stretching, plus the added benefit of breaking down scar tissue and adhesions within the muscle and its fascia.

The time spent on each area depends on where you feel the most sore and tight. A good general rule is to roll each area a minimum of 10 to 15 times. If you have trouble areas or "hot spots," these areas will need more attention. We recommend that when you find these "hot spots," you apply pressure for 20 to 30 seconds to break up the knots.

Use it Often

We recommend using a foam roller, lacrosse ball, or stick even on the days that you are not working out to relieve some of the soreness. You should spend a little extra time addressing problem areas. Foam rolling is one of the most important parts of working out because it can dramatically improve the quality and length of your muscles. It may be painful at first, and you may not want to do it. But it will get easier if you do it consistently. In just a few sessions, you will notice an improvement in your workouts as well as reduced muscle soreness.

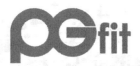

Soft Tissue Work – SMFR & Foam Rolling

Calves	Lats
	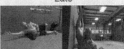
IT Band	Teres Major & Minor
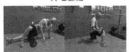	
TFL	Upper Back
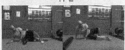	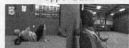
Hamstrings	Mid Back & Thoracic Decompression
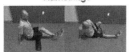	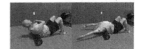
Adductors	Lower Back
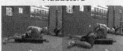	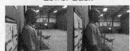
Glute Medius & Piriformis	Pec Minor Major
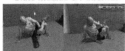	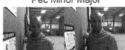
Quadricep	Anterior Delts
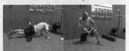	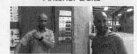
Hip Flexors	Triceps/Biceps
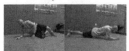	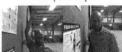
Glute Max	Forearm
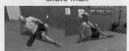	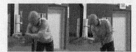

Corrective Exercises

There are specific exercises that can help you overcome any motor dysfunctions or muscle imbalances you may have. These should be performed after you have done your soft tissue or myofascial work with the foam roller, lacrosse ball, or stick. As part of an assessment at PG Fit, we can determine where your tight and weak muscles are and can structure a corrective exercise strategy for you. The charts below provide an example of the type of corrective exercises included in a typical program.

PGfit

Corrective Exercises

FMS (Exercise)	SMFR (Tissue Quality)	Mobility Corrective 1	Activation Corrective 2	Integration Corrective 3
Yellow Active Straight Leg Raise	Calves Hamstrings Hip Flexor TFL Quadriceps Adductors	Leg Lowering	Floor Bridge	PVC Hip Hinge
White Shoulder Mobility	Lats Teres Upper Back Lower Back Chest	T Drill	Band Pull Apart	Standing Cobra
Orange Rotary Stability	Glutes Hip Flexor TFL Lats/Teres Upper Back Mid Back Adductors	Deadbug	Birddog	Pulsed Plank
Red Torso Stability Push Up	Glutes Hip Flexor TFL Lats/Teres Upper Back Mid Back Adductors	Handwalk	Inchworm	Push Up
Blue In-Line Lunge	Glutes Hip Flexor TFL Lats/Teres Upper Back Mid Back Adductors	Pulsed Hip Flexor Mob	Leg Lock Bridge	Split Squat
Green Hurdle Step	Glutes Hip Flexor TFL Lats/Teres Upper Back Mid Back Adductors Quadriceps	Single Leg Balance	Knee Grabs	Mountain Climbers
Purple Deep Squat	Glutes Hip Flexor TFL Lats/Teres Upper Back Mid Back Adductors Quadriceps	Butterfly	Sumo Squat	Air Squat

Static Stretches

At the end of a workout, you should follow a static stretching program to elongate your muscles and help them get back to their proper length-tension relationship. Static means that you hold the stretch in a still or isolated position for at least 20 to 30 seconds. The charts below provide an example of the type of static stretches you should do after a workout.

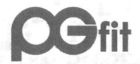

Lengthen Muscle Groups (Static Stretches)

Calves	**Lumbar & Thoracic Extension**
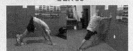	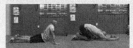
Hamstring	**Lateral Flexion**
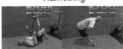	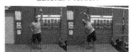
TFL & IT Band	**Shoulder Rotator Cuff**
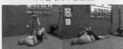	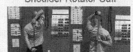
Glute Medius & Piriformis	**Supraspinatus**
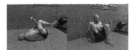	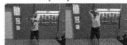
Hip Flexor	**Lats & Posterior Delts**
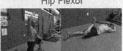	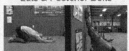
Quadriceps	**Chest & Anterior Delts**
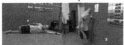	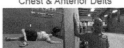
Butterfly & Adductor	**Triceps/Biceps**
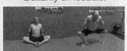	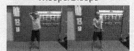
Gluteal	**Wrist**
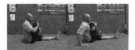	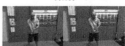
Lumbar Rotation	**Neck**
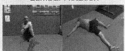	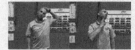

Corrective Exercise Program

I have provided you with a corrective exercise form below so you can see how we structure a flexibility program for our clients. First, we review and check off the soft tissue work (foam rolling exercises) they should be doing when they first come into the gym. Then, we encourage them to lengthen, activate, and integrate their muscles by going through the corrective exercises in the middle section. The first two sections (foam rolling exercises and corrective exercises) should be done prior to working out.

When these are done, clients can go through their structured workout for the day. At the end of their workout, we have them go through the third section of the form where they do static stretches.

Any exercise program you begin should include a flexibility program (soft tissue work, corrective exercises, and stretching). If not, you should question the integrity of the program. By not following these basic foundational principles, you are just setting yourself up to get injured or hurt.

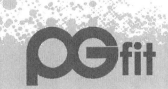

CORRECTIVE EXERCISE
PROGRAM

Name: Date:

Soft Tissue Work (Foam Rolling)

Lower Body	Upper Body
Calves	Lats
IT Band	Teres
TFL	Upper Back
Hamstrings	Mid Back
Adductors	Lower Back
Piriformis	Chest
Quadriceps	Anterior Delts
Hip Flexor	Triceps/Biceps
Glutes	Forearm

Lengthen, Activate & Integrate Muscle Groups

Functional Movement Screen	Color	Lengthen	Activate	Integrate
Active Straight Leg Raise	Yellow	Leg Lowering	Floor Bridge	Good Morning
Shoulder Mobility	White	T Drill	Band Pull Aparts	Standing Cobra
Rotary Stability	Orange	Deadbug	Birddog	Pulsed Planks
Torso Stability Push Up	Red	Hand Walks	Inchworm	Push Up
In-Line Lunge	Blue	Pulsed Hip Flexor Mobs	Leg Lock Bridge	Split Squat
Hurdle Step	Green	SL Balance	Knee Grabs	Mountain Climber
Deep Squat	Purple	Butterfly	Sumo Squats	Air Squats

Static Stretches

Lower Body	Upper Body
Calves (gastroc &soleus)	Lumbar & Thoracic Extension
90/90 Hamstring	Lateral Flexion
TFL & IT Band	Shoulder Rotator Cuff
Piriformis	Supraspinatus
Kneeling Hip Flexor	Lats & Posterior Delts
Side Lying Quadricep	90/90 Chest & Anterior Delts
Butterfly & Adductor	Triceps/Biceps
Gluteal	Wrist
Lumbar Rotation	Neck

The Perfectible Workout

I have also developed a unique resistance training program and fitness level system called The Perfectible Workout. The Perfectible Workout is a workout program and fitness testing system that you can do on your own to lose weight the right way and monitor your progress.

It is one of the most efficient ways to work out. Each time you go through the program, you will be closer to perfecting it and completing a fitness level. By focusing on each stage and phase of training, you will learn how to stabilize and strengthen your body and create power. The variations in this program have the added benefit of keeping your body from physiologically adapting to the workouts, and you will be able to progress from one level to the next.

You will also be able to perfect the plan by learning how to work effectively through all seven movement patterns to overcome your motor dysfunctions and muscle imbalances.

And finally, you'll learn how to incorporate a component called active rest into your program. This allows you to enjoy the maximum benefits of cardiorespiratory training while you are doing resistance training.

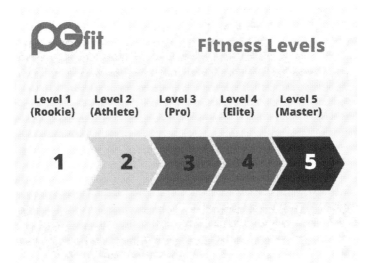

CHAPTER 8
Coaching

When you hear the word "coach," what do you think of? If you've had an opportunity to work with a coach on a sports team, that person probably comes to mind. If you haven't, you might think of a coach as a drill sergeant or a person holding a whistle, yelling at you to run another lap. I had several coaches like that, and I never felt encouraged or motivated to do what they asked of me.

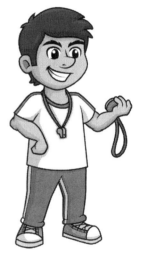

When I think of the word coach, I think of one of the diving coaches I had my first year of college at the University of Hawaii. If you've ever seen the movie *Karate Kid,* Mr. Miyagi was the spitting image of my UH diving coach, Wally Nakamoto. In fact, Wally Nakamoto and the actor that played Mr. Miyagi, Pat Morita, were friends and lived near each other.

My coach, Wally, taught me more about life than diving. He could come across as very arrogant and prideful, but he was one of the best diving coaches in the country. And when I got to know him, he was actually one of the most loving and understanding people I'd ever met.

He taught me the importance of commitment and discipline and that the key to success was consistency and perseverance. He took the time to mentor me and to help me become the best version of myself.

Although I struggled with him at first, he became a great mentor of mine. Even though Wally is no longer with us, I still think about him every once in a while, and the impact he had on my life.

The word coach is an old English word that came from the word stagecoach. A stagecoach was attached to a team of horses and was the primary form of transportation before automobiles were invented. The old English word for coach means "to take you somewhere." A coach takes you somewhere you want to go that you can't get to by yourself.

Coaching is the fifth fundamental of health and fitness. We all need help from time to time. Even the best athletes in the world have several coaches and highly trained professionals they work with to help them become the very best at what they do. There's a reason why celebrities and other highly successful people use coaches and trainers: it works!

It's estimated that about 90 percent of people who start a fitness program will stop before their new routine even becomes a habit. And more than 60 percent quit in the first week. Why? One of the reasons is that it's not easy to change your lifestyle. The media makes it seem like anyone can lose weight and transform their body in a short amount of time if they pick the right program, supplement, gym, etc. But the reality is that getting fit requires a dramatic lifestyle shift that takes determination, support, and a fair amount of time. If any of these components is missing, success becomes less likely.

Everyone needs a coach. But training is not the same thing as coaching. Anyone can work with a personal trainer to count their sets and reps, but is that coaching? No, it's not! Unfortunately, coaches aren't born; they're made. You don't become a coach overnight. It takes time!

I believe that coaching is the most important job in the world. If you think about it, we are all coaches to some degree. If you have children, you know what I'm talking about. Parenting is one of the most significant examples of coaching.

Coaches don't always get it right. There are a lot of good and bad ones out there. I'm sure your parents didn't always get it right, or you didn't always get it right as a parent. But a great coach will believe in you before you start believing in yourself. They will see you as you cannot yet see yourself. Even though you might make mistakes, a great coach will help you become the best version of yourself!

A coach is going to review and measure your progress—that which can be measured can be improved. One of the most important jobs of coaching is ensuring accountability. A coach isn't always going to tell you that you're doing a good job. Sometimes they are going to have difficult conversations with you, especially when you are not making progress.

A coach is going to help you overcome challenges or setbacks. And guess what? At some point, you will have challenges or setbacks. A coach is going to help you focus on one percent improvement every day. If you can start improving one percent every day, within a matter of months, you can see some pretty drastic and remarkable changes. Just imagine if you improved one percent every day for an entire year!

Did you know that a personal trainer doesn't even have to be certified to call themselves a personal trainer? In the fitness industry, you don't have to have a certification to work with the human body. You need a license to offer manicures, pedicures, or to cut hair, but you don't need one to train the human body. You don't even need to have a certification to call yourself a nutrition consultant or nutritionist.

There are a number of personal trainers out there who can train you or tell you what to eat. But to be a fitness professional, you need to have certifications and experience. I recommend that every personal trainer have at least three basic certifications before they start working on specializations. They should be certified as a personal trainer and also have both nutrition and biomechanical certifications from a nationally recognized institution. The first certified personal trainer certification that I received was from an organization that is still considered very reputable, but it only took me a couple of hours to take an open book exam to get certified. Anyone can call themselves a personal trainer!

One of the greatest recognitions a fitness professional can have is to be called a coach. Coaches are made, and it takes time to become a great coach. A coach is a mentor—someone who's going to help you get from where you are to where you want to be. A coach is going to focus on the fundamentals of health and fitness to help you lose weight the right way.

Hopefully, you now understand that you need a personal trainer—and more importantly, a coach—to help you with your health and fitness journey. We all need help from time to time. Heck, I work with a personal trainer too. I don't need someone to design my program, but I need to be motivated and held accountable like everyone else.

Now that you know you need a personal trainer, just like I do, take a moment to fill out the form below. Write down three expectations that you have for your trainer/coach.

Three Expectations for My Coach

• _____

• _____

• _____

I would encourage you to look for a personal trainer in your area to help you address the fundamentals of health and fitness, so you can lose weight the right way. Be honest with them about your goals and expectations.

Remember, a personal trainer should not only have credentials and experience but should also be a coach. A coach will believe in you, see you for who you are capable of becoming, and help you become the best version of yourself.

CHAPTER 9

Service

This book has taught you a system and program that will help you lose weight the right way so that you can become the healthiest you have been in years. The system is called the Five Fundamentals of Health and Fitness. Hopefully, you have taken notes and completed the exercises at the end of each chapter so that you will be well on your way to making the Five Fundamentals a way of life.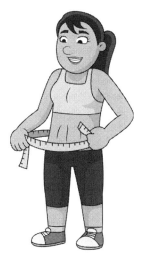

By following these basics, you have learned there is a right way and a wrong way to lose weight. You understand that you need to focus on your health in order to become fit. You also need to achieve balance and moderation on your health and fitness journey. I have witnessed so many people lose weight the wrong way, and I am sure you have too. I have also watched many clients reach their health and fitness goals the right way, but then eventually revert back to their old habits and gain the weight back.

Why? In order for your results to become part of your lifestyle, you will have to set an example for those around you and help empower them to achieve their own health and fitness goals. This is why the last statements on the Five Fundamentals Quiz relate to using your newfound knowledge to empower those around you. The best way to find yourself is to lose yourself in the service to others.

It's one thing to take care of or help others, and it's another thing to serve them. When we take care of or help others, we oftentimes enable them. As a parent, we must take care of our children when they are young to provide for their basic necessities, but as our children become older and more mature, they need to take responsibility for their own actions. Enabling has the effect of releasing the person from having to take responsibility for their own actions.

The first few years I worked as a personal trainer, I thought I was helping my clients by telling them what to do to reach their health and fitness goals. Instead, I enabled them by allowing them to use excuses for why they weren't successful. They would have moderate success losing weight, but most of them would gain the weight back after they stopped training.

When we serve one another, we help them by doing work for them without expecting anything else in return. We accept the person for who they are, even their shortcomings and imperfections. We learn to be patient, understanding, and tolerant of the decisions they make. We can also serve them by setting an example for the way they should live their lives.

Service can be difficult, especially when it comes to family members and friends because they are often the ones who contributed to your bad habits, poor health, and fitness choices. Once you take ownership of the choices and decisions you have made, you will be able to develop the right habits and behaviors that will help you make the necessary lifestyle changes for long-term success.

It will be easier to see past your family members' and friends' shortcomings or imperfections and meet them where they are on their own health and fitness journey. You will be able to lead by example. With a servant-like attitude, you will be patient, understanding, and tolerant of the decisions they make, regardless of whether it affects you or not. You will yearn for them to be healthy and fit, and you will want to serve them. You will be able to help them make positive changes in their health and fitness, and empower them to help others do the same.

I know this to be true, because I have seen this with my clients, my wife, and my son, and I am starting to see it with my family and my in-laws. I have seen them start to make some positive changes in their health and fitness because of my example and my passion for serving them. I'm not perfect, and I still fall short at times. But the point is to keep trying and persevere.

I'm going to tell you again that there is no diet, magic pill, or specific workout routine that is going to help you lose weight and keep it off for good. It's going to take a lot of hard work. You are going to have to be dedicated. You are going to have to get used to being uncomfortable. Until you're sick of being sick and tired, nothing is going to change.

If you've ever flown in a plane, you've heard the flight attendant repeat that if the cabin pressure drops during the flight, you're instructed to put on your own oxygen mask before helping others. If you don't, you will lose oxygen, stop breathing, and possibly die. You can't help others until you help yourself.

You have to start by working on your own health and fitness, but once you start to develop the right habits, behaviors, and lifestyle changes to have long-term success, you can start to help others do the same. Remember, the only way for you to have long-term success is to help those around you do the same. It is my hope that you will be able to take the principles and teachings I have shared with you in this book and apply them to your own lives, and then empower others to do the same!

CHAPTER 10

Testimonials

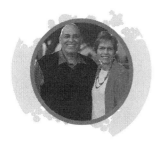

I had toyed with the idea of participating in a PG Fit event when it was offered at St. John. Due to my own inertia and calendar conflicts, I was able to attend only the third session. How I wish I had started when it all began. This is due to two important factors:

1. The assessment process is extensive and very helpful. I learned there was much more to it than weighing and measuring. They also assessed balance, flexibility, and other key physical criteria. That information is used to tailor a program that accounts for individual variations in strength and ability.

2. The trainers at PG Fit are extremely knowledgeable, gracious, helpful, encouraging, and patient. I look forward to every (well almost every!) workout with them. They challenge me but also know how to spur me on and help me make great progress. We are building a culture of health at St. John Lutheran Church in part due to our connection with PG Fit.

– DAVID B.

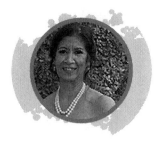

I'm so very glad I went to PG Fit and started my fitness journey. I had not been consistent with an exercise program for over 15 years, but once I tried their free introductory class, I was hooked. I really like that they genuinely care about the whole aspect of my fitness: exercise, nutrition, and coaching. They give an initial fitness assessment that lets them know which exercises are appropriate in order to avoid injury and to progress to the next level of exercises. I came in with constant sciatica pain on both sides of my lower back. Since I began doing the rolling, stretching, and exercises they taught me, my pain has been gone! I have been working with PG Fit for two years now, and I still absolutely love the variety of circuit training exercises they lead us through, as well as their coaching and the continual daily encouragement and teachings on exercises and nutrition.

– Linda W.

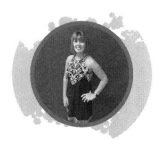

I joined PG Fit at age 47. My goal at the time was just to fit back into my clothes. When I started, I ran about three times a week (training for a half marathon) and lifted weights at the gym. My first couple of months with PG Fit were fun. I met a lot of great people and most of them were within ten years of my age and were fighting the same battles as me. I've lost 15 pounds in six months. It may not seem like a lot to you, but I did it on my terms … not some crazy "lose weight fast" scam. I lost fat and gained muscle. I did it with great coaches who constantly changed the workouts, new friends who shared the same goals, new knowledge about nutrition and supplements, and a new habit that I'm glad I acquired … the need and WANT to work out! Good luck with your journey! I hope that you get an addiction like mine!

– Lisa B.

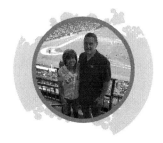

About a year and a half ago, my wife Tracie and I were looking for a place to help us reach our fitness goals. Fortunately, we found PG Fit. At the time, I was very overweight with poor balance and flexibility. I was taking medication for high blood pressure and had pain and stiffness in my joints. Michael and his team have helped me to lose weight and improve my balance and flexibility as well as my physical stamina and strength. My doctors have been impressed with the changes, and they have taken me off of some of my prescriptions. And my joint pain has been reduced considerably. I will keep working with Michael and his team to continue to improve my fitness with the goal of eliminating my medications altogether.

– KYLE & TRACIE S.

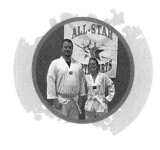

Everybody has excuses. And I was no different. Too tired, too busy, too early, too late. Add the medical excuses on top of those—four surgeries that removed most of the cartilage from both knees, two lower back surgeries for herniated discs, and Parkinson's disease—and you get me ... at nearly 300 pounds. I had almost given up on ever being able to do anything "athletic" again. Just getting out of bed took 30 minutes. Stairs? Forget it. Running? Not even in my vocabulary. I had gotten this stupid idea of joining a gym, thinking it would magically transform me into the shape I was when I graduated from college.

It took about a month or two to get enough courage to walk into the gym. My first class was with Michael. I remember when I was about 10 minutes into it and thought I might just collapse on the mat and die. We had just finished doing goblin squats, and Michael smiles and says, "Ok. Good warmup. Now for the workout." If I could have moved my legs at that point, I might have just walked out and given up.

Then Michael started explaining each part of the workout and key movements. Everything he was explaining sounded like Charlie Brown's teacher talking, but somehow, I managed to get through the class. As I'm dragging myself out of the gym, Michael gives me a high five and says, "You made it. It will be easier tomorrow." I went back the next day and made it through another class. The more I went to class, the more Charlie Brown's teacher turned into my life-changing coach, Michael.

It's been a little over a year and a half since I started, and I've lost 40 pounds of fat—just fat. But the weight loss is only a small part of PG Fit. Nutrition, hydration, stabilization, strength, and power are all incorporated into 45 minutes a day. I'm now in the best shape I've been in 20 years. I'm able to run five miles in the morning and still have a normal day. I actually look forward to 5:00 a.m. because I can go to the gym.

About 90 percent of my office coworkers go to the same CrossFit gym. Every day, I hear how someone has hurt their back or some other part. That doesn't happen at PG Fit. Every trainer actually knows what they are talking about, and they pay attention to how your body moves. I could write pages of good things PG Fit has done to help improve my life, but I'll sum it up by saying, "Try it. You will be hooked."

– Toby K.

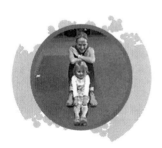

I began training with PG Fit during my third trimester of pregnancy with my third child. I had been working with a private trainer for about three years who had recently quit training. I was looking for a gym with group training, thinking I just needed to keep an appointment to hold me accountable to a workout so I could "stay in shape."

I was pleasantly surprised that I received so much more than I expected when I began training at PG Fit! I found a training environment that held me accountable because of an appointment, and they wanted to help me not only meet but exceed my fitness goals.

PG Fit has a very supportive and helpful approach that fits my busy schedule. I have been at PG Fit for four years now, and I have seen improvement in so many areas. My form and mechanics have improved, as well as my diet and the diet of my family. I have been coached on effective nutrition and supplement use. I have gained the amount of muscle I wanted without being or looking bulky. I lost my pregnancy weight within a few months of returning to the gym postpartum (after a congratulatory and supportive call from the owner). I am in the best shape of my life—even after having three children and working a full-time job the entire journey. In addition, I have made some new friends and found a supportive community at PG Fit.

– MICHELLE P.

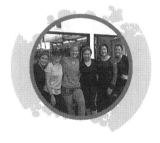

PG Fit has been a great place to help me become my best self. I have learned so many things about living a healthy lifestyle and having a healthy body through my training there. Nutrition, cardio endurance, strength training, and flexibility are only a few of the concepts I have learned to incorporate in my daily life.

Every aspect is important, and PG Fit covers them all daily—it's much more than just going to a gym to work out. The information I am given educates me regarding all areas of fitness, not just one. The support system of the training staff and other clients in the group fitness classes helps hold me accountable. It helps me achieve my small daily goals as well as the long-term goals set within the program. PG Fit has given me a solid foundation to build a healthy lifestyle each and every day. Thanks, PG Fit!!!

– TRICIA M.

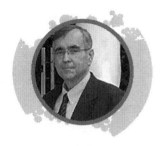

I joined PG Fit back in December 2016, after being encouraged by my wife, Linda, to try one of their promotional offers. Michael performed my initial assessment, and I started going to the 5:00 a.m. Personal Group Trainer sessions twice a week. After a short time, I was hooked on going and started a regular routine with the 5:00 a.m. crowd, twice a week. And by early spring 2017, I was going three times a week.

The thing I really like about PG Fit is the positive and supportive environment—not only the staff but with other members too. In addition to an emphasis on physical training, there is equal emphasis on proper nutrition, water intake, and offsite cardio.

I also want to thank Michael and the team for the vast number of PG Fit exercise and nutritional videos available on YouTube and Facebook. They are very beneficial.

As we approach the end of 2018, I'm still participating with the 5:00 a.m. crowd and continually look forward to my three-times-a-week workout. Michael, Seth, and Kelsey are a great training staff and take a sincere interest in helping you advance in the areas of physical strength and endurance. And they are always checking in to see how you're doing.

I truly feel much better now than I have in many years, and I'm looking forward to more years working with the PG Fit Team to improve my physical strength, nutrition, hydration, and cardio exercising.

Thank you, PG Fit!!!

– MARK W.

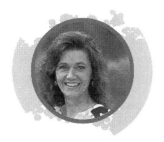

I've never been a gym person. I hated the idea of paying for "fitness" when all I thought I needed was a pair of running shoes and some awesome trails! The personal trainer aspect of PG Fit has totally changed my mind as well as improved my overall fitness. The sessions have a different focus every month and provide different exercises each day—no boring, repeating routines!

The trainers help me improve my form and ensure I do everything correctly. If I can't perform a move correctly, the trainers personalize my workout with another exercise until I'm strong enough for the full move. While stretching at the end of each workout, the trainers provide educational talks on subjects like nutrition, cardio, supplements, resistance training, and coaching. They encourage excellent nutrition and send many recipes that are delicious and doable. PG Fit is a one-stop-shop for all fitness needs.

– TAMI M.

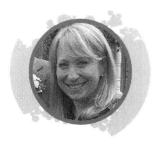

I love working out with PG Fit because it is always a challenging workout that works my entire body. I appreciate that the trainers make sure I am using proper form—which decreases my chances of injury and forced downtime while accelerating my results. While staying fit is important to me, regular and consistent exercise with a personal trainer really helps keep my anxiety and depression in check too. I love my PG Fit "family!"

– AMY P.

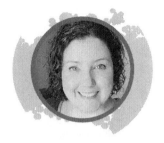

I've had three lower back surgeries. The first came after doing a popular "boot camp" for two months. The second came after I hired a trainer to come to my home—a trainer I hired to teach me how to strengthen my core to support my injured back.

At that point, I didn't think anyone could help me. And that's when I found PG Fit. From day one, I was never told to do an exercise that was too advanced for me, nor was I told to "keep going" even if I couldn't maintain proper form. (In case it's not clear, these are the techniques which led to my injuries.)

I wanted someone knowledgeable about nutrition and exercise, and someone to hold me accountable. PG Fit has given me so much more than that!

I never thought I would be able to work out and get results without being in constant pain. Now, I'm excited about the progress I'm making, and I rarely have pain!

Michael and Seth are amazing trainers with a wealth of knowledge and determination to do what's right for each of their clients. It's not about "ten more reps;" it's about doing them the right way, so you work the proper muscles and prevent injuries. #ProudToBePGFit

– KAREN R.

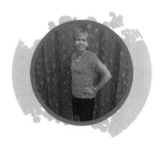

After turning 60, I developed some arthritis in my hip and some lower back disc problems, which translated to chronic pain. Not wanting to lose mobility, I joined a gym. The trainer there just showed me how to use the machines. I had a hard time staying motivated and didn't really know if I was helping or hurting myself. After breaking my ankle on a hike and completing PT, I knew I needed something more.

I had seen my husband's energy and movement improve remarkably after personal training with Michael at PG Fit, so I decided to give it a try. I was surprised at the extent of the initial assessment and how personalized the training sessions were, based on my physical needs and fitness. The personal training helped me improve my strength and conditioning and also lowered my pain level. I was able to reduce the amount of medication I took. I was also better able to help with my young and active grandchildren, which was a huge plus!

Eventually, I progressed enough to join the group class at PG Fit. There again, the exercises are adjusted according to individual levels, so there is space for improvement with less fear of injury. Better yet, the group dynamic provides encouragement and motivation. We have a lot of fun together in the group and with the trainers. The basic exercises can be done anywhere, which is really helpful because I travel frequently and can continue with a basic workout wherever I go.

I have also benefited from the nutritional instruction at PG Fit and the emphasis on goal-setting. I have been able to lower my body fat percentage, keep my pain medication at a minimum, increase my fitness and endurance, fit better into my clothes, and generally feel better. The combination of healthy eating and exercise has helped improve my blood pressure, cholesterol, and bone density. I am very thankful for the trainers and all the folks at PG Fit!

– DIANE B.

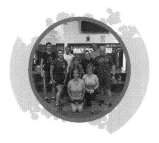

In my experience, trainers are either really knowledgeable about designing good workout programs, great at motivating you during workouts, or skilled at teaching you about nutrition. They are almost never good at all three.

The best thing I have found about PG Fit is their staff actually check all three boxes. No matter your physical background or goals, their well-rounded expertise increases your chance of success. This is critical. Many people put out the necessary effort to get in shape, but unfortunately, they lack the proper knowledge. Therefore, they fail. PG Fit provides that knowledge in a friendly, positive environment.

– CHRIS P.

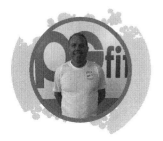

I am a male in my late 50s, and I have been a customer at PG Fit for three and a half years. I attend the group workouts 2–3 times per week and try to play tennis twice a week. My body fat has been reduced by about half during my time at PG Fit. My weight loss has been significant, but more importantly, I have traded fat for muscle through the diet and exercise program at PG Fit. Michael Romig and his staff offer the complete solution we all need for nutrition, strength training, flexibility, structured cardio programs, and professional advice—all tailored to individual needs. PG Fit has a group of professionals with certifications to prove it, and they offer a better approach and environment than what's available at commercial gyms. For me, it has been long-term lifestyle change at its best.

– GREG B.

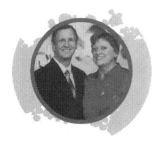

The results were amazing. I began training mainly for health reasons, but the bonus was how great I felt and looked. What I mean by amazing is that I went from a size 18 to an 8. I have more energy and feel healthier in a short amount of time. Michael has always combined food intake education with workouts. This is a win-win situation. I cannot say how grateful I am to have the PG Fit trainers for my workouts.

– SELMA H.

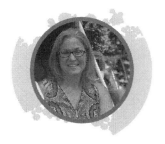

I've been a member at PG Fit for more than five years. I take the group classes and have regular sessions with a personal trainer. Personal training has helped me become a better planner and be accountable for my results. I've been able to gain muscle and lose body fat while seeing results on the scale. It's always easy to let life get the better of you, but at PG Fit, they are always there to keep you going!

– Lesli C.

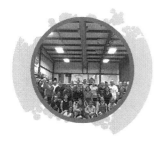

I started the PG Fit program after seeing the results of a friend. My goal at the time was to lose a few pounds and to lead a healthier lifestyle. I had tried many exercise and dieting programs over the years, none lasting more than a few months. Two years after joining PG Fit, I'm down to my high school weight. I've lost my muffin top and about a third of my body fat. At 55, I feel stronger than ever.

I've also learned more balanced, healthy, and sustainable eating habits. The key to this program for me: the instructors are encouraging, caring, and fun; the workouts are directed and constantly changing so I don't get bored; and the small class sizes enable more personalized instruction and camaraderie. Maybe most importantly for me, I was not expected to change everything at once. I continue to make gradual improvements to my eating and fitness habits with the help of weekly information and tips from the trainers.

– Laurie H.

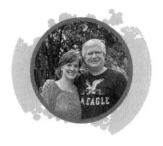

I have learned so much about working out, eating better, and living a healthier lifestyle. I am happy to say that I have lost 37 pounds, have never felt better, and always look forward to my gym days! Without the help of the PG Fit trainers, this would not have been possible. I am blessed to share my story with others and have friends that have not only joined me at the gym in person but also via Facebook during the detox challenges. Thank you, PG Fit, for making a difference in my life!!

– BECKY B.

I had struggled with my weight my entire life. It was never really bad (I never let it go over 160 pounds at the height of 5'8"), but it was not good either. I had times when I lost 20 pounds. But in addition to feeling weak and terrible from starving myself, I would gain it back immediately after going back to eating normally. I used to work out regularly, but my body never showed the work I put in it. After doing CrossFit for a couple of months, my knee and my shoulder gave up, which led me to a point where I felt I needed help.

I found PG Fit online, and after a hesitation phase of a couple of weeks, I went for it and made an appointment. The first assessment with Michael was an eye-opener for me in so many ways. He immediately saw my weaknesses, and for the first time, I felt there was someone who could help me get fit and strong without hurting my knee and shoulder. The first assessment also included a weigh-in on the impedance scale. My results were 158 pounds and 35 percent body fat. I felt terrible and was eager to start.

Today, I am down almost 30 pounds, and my body fat is around 19 percent. I don't want to lose any more weight, but I'm still working on my body composition. I'm doing 3–4 sessions of resistance training and two cardio sessions per week. I am currently on macros that equal

1,750 calories/day, but my final goal is to have my body live healthily on 2,300–2,500 calories/day without gaining weight.

Thank you, PG Fit, Michael, and Seth. Your expertise, friendship, and encouragement have helped me change my life. You not only worked with me to become fit but also helped me understand that being fit and healthy is something you have to commit to every single day!

– JANA K.

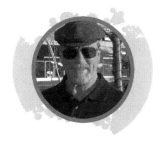

I am a 74-year-old retired military officer who joined PG Fit in December 2017. By virtue of having spent 30 years in the army and almost 20 years after that in the defense industry, I have been almost continuously involved in some form of workout regimen—formal or informal—all of my life. **PG Fit is, without a doubt, the best all-around fitness program with which I have been involved in all of that time!** Let me tell you briefly why I think so …

Professional. The staff at PG Fit is personable, friendly, approachable, knowledgeable, well-trained, and experienced. They are patient and never disparaging. Working with them is actually an enjoyable experience because the atmosphere is one of striving for personal improvement and never one of unwanted competition or intimidation. The staff helps you get you better!

Comprehensive. The program stresses the critical importance of understanding the link between nutrition and exercise. The staff is well-trained in the nutritional aspects of fitness and constantly emphasizes the necessity of managing the body across the spectrum of fitness. Workouts target the entire body, are very well designed, and absolutely never boring. There is ample individual attention in the group workouts, and personal training is available if desired.

Adaptable. Everyone gets a good workout! Significantly different fitness levels can, and often do, work out together. And due to the experience of the staff and the design of the workouts, everyone works to his/her individual fitness requirements.

As you can no doubt tell, I am a believer in the PG Fit program. Regardless of where one is on the fitness/nutrition spectrum, becoming a member will result in a positive and productive experience.

– Doug S.

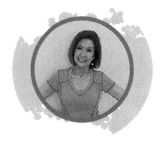

I have always enjoyed exercising, and I've tried a variety of workouts such as ballet, kickboxing, hot yoga, reformer Pilates, and Jazzercise. Our metabolism slows as we age, causing muscle loss and fat gain. PG Fit has been the "best fit" for me to decelerate that process. The difference has been the individual fitness evaluation and instruction that a personal trainer provides. From the beginning, Michael emphasized the importance of wearing a heart rate monitor to more efficiently track our target zones and improve our cardiovascular endurance. The wrist bands are helpful in identifying muscle imbalances and range of motion deficiencies. Stretching out with foam rollers before class and after with bands warms up muscles and smooths out knots. This form of self-massage has been an invaluable practice for me that enhances the quality of each 45-minute workout.

When a state-of-the-art fitness center opened nearby with its numerous machines, classes, saunas, and pools, I tried it. In no time, however, I returned to PG Fit because of its excellent trainers. They modify and tailor every exercise for each of us, as needed, to prevent injury, and they periodically reassess our flexibility and balance. I have been able to track my progress on the electronic screen during sessions and with the provided app when on the go, which has continually motivated me to improve.

In almost two years of PG Fit membership, I have lost 14 pounds and 8 percent body fat. I have also increased my OwnIndex fitness score by 14 points. The score and weight loss have been added benefits to my main goal of gaining strength and maintaining balance and flexibility. This IS the best I have felt in years. I appreciate the professionalism, creativity, patience, and fun that Michael, Seth, and Kelsey bring to the gym.

– THERESA J.

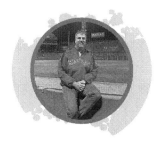

When I first started working out at PG Fit, I lost 18 pounds of fat and gained 5 pounds of lean muscle. A year later, I was diagnosed with brain cancer and told that I would only have a year to live. Four years later, I am still working out at PG Fit, and I am grateful for each and every day I have. I currently take medication for seizures which prevents me from coming into the gym sometimes, but I work out in the group classes a few days a week. I am so thankful that I am able to work out and focus on my health and fitness!

– SEAN S.

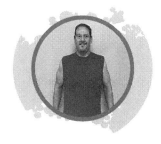

Thanks to life's challenges, I needed to start a training program. I'm so glad I found PG Fit. I have lost over 40 pounds of fat so far! What an amazing experience to know it can be done! These past several months have been life-changing, and with the help and knowledge of personal trainers truly giving it their all for me, I am achieving my goals. Thanks for your dedication. I will always be grateful.

– ALEX P.

Thank You

I would like to thank you for taking the time to read this instructional book and for your commitment to your health and fitness goals. If you have read this book and completed the exercises at the end of each chapter, you are well on your way to accomplishing your health and fitness goals the right way.

As we discussed in the final chapter, service is the most important element of your success long term. Anyone can lose weight, but can they do it the right way and empower others to do the same? I would recommend that you start by inviting your family members and friends to read this book. Help them begin their own health and fitness journey and encourage them to go to the gym with you. Hopefully, you will invite them to be part of the PG Fit family by participating in the 28-Day Challenge on the next page!

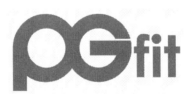

PGFit.com
14405 Telge Road
Cypress, TX 77429
(832) 303-7004
Facebook.com/PGFit

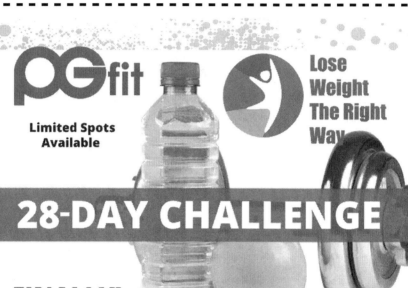

About the Author

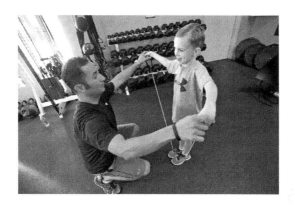

Michael is a master trainer, author, wellness consultant, speaker, and the owner of PG FIT. He is a certified and accredited personal trainer and nutritionist who has helped hundreds of clients reach their health and fitness goals.

Michael is currently pursuing a Doctorate in Health Science. He received a Master's in Business Administration, a Master of Science in Exercise Science & Health Promotion, and a Bachelor of Science in Psychology. He holds several nationally recognized personal training certifications through accredited organizations such as NASM, NCSF, PFIT, NFPT, NSCA, CrossFit, FMS, TRX, USAW, Cooper, and ISSA.

He also has seven advanced specializations in nutrition, PEMF, corrective exercise, performance enhancement training, rehabilitative exercise training, physical therapy, and strength and conditioning.

Michael is a member of AAU and USA Diving and an All-American and national champion. He is married and has an eighteen-year-old son who is also a diver at Princeton. He enjoys running, mountain biking, playing golf, and the occasional weekend skydiving.

You can learn more about Michael and his personal training studio at PGFIT.com

Made in the USA
Columbia, SC
26 February 2025

54483723R00080